BE THERE

My Lived Experience
with My Sister's Bipolar Disorder

LINSEY WILLIS

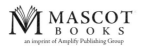

For more information, please contact:
Mascot Books, an imprint of Amplify Publishing Group
620 Herndon Parkway, Suite 220
Herndon, VA 20170
info@mascotbooks.com

Library of Congress Control Number: 2023915713

CPSIA Code: PRV0524A

ISBN-13: 978-1-63755-928-4

Printed in the United States

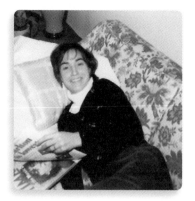
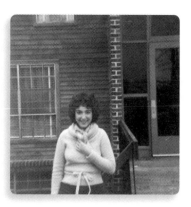
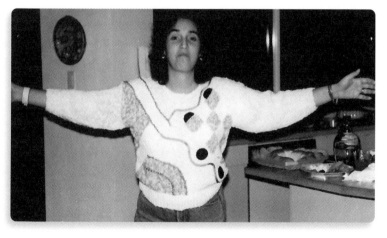

This book is dedicated to my sister, Betsy, and to every mentally ill person who is struggling to cope with their illness in a society that stigmatizes them.

It is also dedicated to the family members who live with their loved one's illness and whose pain often goes unnoticed.

CONTENTS

PREFACE

Betsy began a life full of promise. She was beautiful, bright, and a gifted writer. Her devaluation began with an illness labeled *bipolar disorder*. I thought that if she wrote about her life and what she experienced with the disorder (and how it destroyed her hopes and dreams), she would be doing something productive. After the diagnosis she experienced a brief period of time when she was motivated and creative enough to put some of her thoughts on paper. She never completed her written story, despite all our attempts to encourage her. She did not take us up on our offer to buy her a PC, so she could write whenever she felt motivated.

This is the start of my sister's story in her own words:

My name is Betsy Craig. When I was younger I was immensely proud of my name and successes and potential. So much that I refused to change my name during two marriages. But recently it's been all down-hill.

I have had bipolar disorder, manic type, for twenty years, more recently complicated by drug misuse, reckless living, and at least six overdoses. My manic episodes feel like day-long anxiety, with racing thoughts, and most nightmarish, is the insomnia lasting days, exacerbating more intense symptoms.

Then the depression. This comes on suddenly (like a thick black cloud) and is fraught with despondency, low energy, low self-esteem, and thoughts of suicide. The flighty over-blown self-confidence (doctors call it grandiosity) is gone and gives way to tears and inertia.

I had this illness (or it had me) by the age of nineteen when I was in college (SMU now University of Massachusetts, Dartmouth). After hospitalization, diagnosis, treatment, and "stabilization," I finished college and graduate school (University of Pennsylvania) during which times the mood swings flew back and forth with my warped help of throwing away my lithium and anti-depressants—several times.

I've experienced periods of anorexia, bulimia, hypersexuality, kleptomania, and even paranoia. Nevertheless, I was an excellent student and had many friends. The turmoil was private, except to my devoted, very worried parents. This illness affects the whole family; it's heartbreaking and backbreaking.

In addition to my graduate degree (MSW) I also took certification courses in family therapy, substance abuse, and child abuse. Every job I applied for I got and developed into a well-respected and well paid counselor.

- But I couldn't counsel myself!
- Two failed marriages,
- prescriptions drug misuse and abuse,

- occasional use of street drugs and alcohol to combat sleeplessness or depression,
- fifteen hospitalizations in the last twenty years,
- unemployable,
- and, to my mind, not too likeable or loveable.

My name is still Betsy Craig, and there's still the old me at the core, hiding, I think, from the bipolar me. But I'm trying a different self-help route now—living in an adult assisted living facility where I don't have to be alone and lonely; and more importantly, my medications are controlled. I'm still fragile and scared, but I'm determined to achieve intelligent stability.

One final note: Even though I've read that Florida is lagging behind in the field of Mental Health, I've had wonderful doctors who have tried to help me, despite myself. However, in the area of assisted living facilities (other than for the elderly) Florida is a Veritable Wasteland.

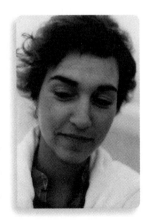

Shortly after Patty Duke published the book *A Brilliant Madness*, my father suggested I, Linsey, read it because it was about her struggle with bipolar disorder. I was surprised because, for so long, he told me he and my mother didn't need the National Alliance for the Mentally Ill (NAMI) and coped quite well on their own. Whatever reading material I sent home, my mother would say he hadn't read it or was reluctant to read it. This attitude was narrow and unsympathetic, considering that the illness was passed down to my sister through his genes. I thought, many times, the least he could have done was make an attempt to learn more about Betsy's struggle with the devastating illness. Over the years, he appeared to try to learn all he could about her illness, but when he approached eighty years of age (October 28, 2005, was his eightieth birthday), his primary thoughts focused on staying healthy (he had cardiopulmonary disease, a.k.a. COPD); taking care of my mother, who was suffering with congestive heart failure; and making plans for the end of his life, which included making sure my sister was taken care of for the rest of her life. Sadly, I lost my mother in July 2006 and my father in October 2007, two weeks shy of his eighty-second birthday. He was blessed to have celebrated his eightieth birthday party with many friends and me.

When this book was in its early draft stages, my father read it, and he said that many of the pages described Betsy and admitted, although reluctantly, that he finally gained insight into her illness and struggles. I was thrilled that he finally started to understand the illness and appeared to be profoundly serious, compassionate, and concerned about her long-term welfare.

I want anyone who is a medical or health professional and is reading this book to understand that I do not write—nor am I presenting myself—as an expert in the field but as a layperson who has had a great deal of experience dealing with my sister's illness.

Prior to my father's death in 2007, I hoped that he would no longer refer to my sister as "loony tunes" or to the short-lived relationships she had with men as "ninety-day wonders." I also hoped he would discontinue his depersonalization of her by ignoring her when she visited them or refusing to visit her with my mother. Both he and my mother lost their desire to see her again after she hit my mother with a shoe because they were afraid to have her in the house. At the time I supported their decision, but was very sad.

After my mother passed away in 2006, my dad asked me to drive him to New Jersey to visit Betsy. My husband and I tried to talk him out of it because I did not want to drive to and from New Jersey; I did not have the time to do so, and I felt strongly that if he visited her in the efficiency apartment and building where she was living (old and dirty carpeting, old and dirty building, etcetera), it would do him more harm than good. I was very sad that he would never see her again. I know this was right.

At that time she was living in the apartment; she was later caught shoplifting and then transferred to a psychiatric hospital in Hackensack, New Jersey. He had not seen her in over nine years!

But as I have learned over the years, such is life when you have a family member with mental illness. An example is a friend from high school whose nephew was a seriously ill paranoid schizophrenic. Based on what I recall being told, he was also paranoid. He would never stay on his medication, and his mother feared him so much that she moved to another state so he would not be able to find her. She finally gave up her long struggle to help him as her years-long attempts to do so failed. I am quite sure there are thousands of families who chose the same route.

I know that there is a great deal of scientific evidence that mental illness is biologically based, and therefore, it is not my father's fault that my sister inherited the disorder. Although for a long time he did not understand her illness and was not as compassionate as he became later on, my father cannot be blamed for causing my sister's disorder.

Dear Linse,

Isn't this pretty stationary? Thankyou so much for your consideration + generosity. I guess it's daddy ... but how does he expect me to get toothpaste, shampoo, why do I have to depend on Drew? I mean it's really nice that he cares but when he calls he's so verbally abusive and sarcastic. His family has tons of money. Oh get this - his oldest sister's

5th husband is Bi Pola he's an aeronautical en + she's a dentist. W decided to come home months for a break they were both doing grass. Well, mummy even sure I can c home for X-mas. What they think I am, a murderer? I've never sa but he is a selfish a bitch: never takes calls. Barbara's pare her come home indefic support in very nice while she takes a 6 mo. tion. Her husband's Ed:

My father, Robert T. Craig, Jr., had a dominant and significant impact on my sister and my life, which is why he is mentioned many times. For example, I believe that his inconsistent behavior toward Betsy was because he could never tell what mood she would be in when she called, and he was also very moody. Subsequently, he responded to her based upon how she behaved. In other words, if she was nasty, he would listen and then terminate the conversation because she continued with her nasty comments and manic behavior. To the left is a letter Betsy wrote to me, which included many negative comments about him.

In the late 1980s, I learned about an organization called the National Alliance for the Mentally Ill (NAMI), and attended a NAMI meeting in Boca Raton, Florida. Initially, I did not realize that mental illnesses were far more common than cancer, diabetes, heart disease, or arthritis or that the National Institute of Mental Health (NIMH) estimated that one out of four families in the United States had a loved one with a mental illness. It was a relief to be advised that mental illnesses are not the result of weak character or bad parenting skills, and to learn that many historical figures who have enriched our lives had mental illnesses. Some who stand out are Vincent van Gogh, Eugene O'Neill, Abraham Lincoln, Ernest Hemingway, Winston Churchill, Isaac Newton, Leo Tolstoy, and Ludwig van Beethoven. It is so unfortunate that this list includes contemporaries such as Anthony Bourdain, the celebrity chef, and Kate Spade, the fashion designer, who both committed suicide. Betsy Ann Craig might have been on this list (I still hold some guilt for not sufficiently encouraging her to write so others could understand). This book is my heartfelt endeavor to share my story about my loving and beautiful and brilliant sister, Betsy, who, in her own way, enriched my life. For example, she helped me to be a better and more generous caregiver. I also learned how to become more patient.

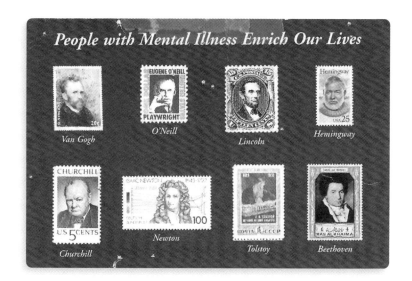

People with Mental Illness Enrich Our Lives

Van Gogh

O'Neill

Lincoln

Hemingway

Churchill

Newton

Tolstoy

Beethoven

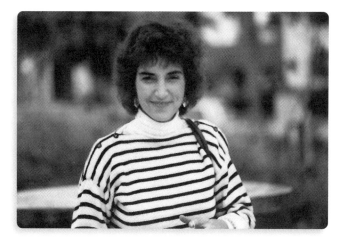

The handwritten letter that follows is an example of Betsy's creative writing and is her message to you and all your family members.

Dear Friends,

Never tell people how to do things.

- Tell them what you want them to achieve and they will surprise you with their ingenuity.

- Patience and perseverance have a magical effect before which difficulties disappear and obstacles vanish.

- Never give up, for that is just the place and time that the tide will turn.

- Work joyfully and peacefully, knowing that right thoughts and right efforts will inevitably bring about right results.

- He who has acheived success has worked well, laughted often and loved much.

- Love is the communion of two hearts.

- Friendship is love and understanding.

- I am a glorious child of God. I am joyful, serene, positive and loving.

- To understand the heart and mind of a person, look not at what he has acheived already, but at what he (she) aspires to do.

Betsy

PRAYER FOR MY SISTER[1]

Together on life's journey, we traveled and shared lots of happy times and many tears, always being there for each other through the years. But my sister went to heaven on September 4 this year (2022), and a dove followed her with a parcel and a cheer. Betsy, be careful when you open it. It's full of beautiful things. Inside are one million hugs to say how much I miss you and now I send you all my love. I will hold you closer than my heart, and there you will remain to walk with me throughout my life until we meet again.

You are now in God's garden, where he found you an empty space. He looked down upon this earth and saw your tired, weary face. He put his arms around you and lifted you to rest, because he knew that since the fire you were in a terrible place. You lost all your possessions, your home, and all your friends. He also knew you would never be the same or well again.

If sunflowers grow in heaven, Lord, please pick a bunch for me. Place them in my sister's arms and tell her they're from me. Tell her that I love and miss her, and when she turns to smile, place a kiss upon her cheek and hold her for a while.

Because remembering her is easy, as I do every day, but there is an empty spot in my heart that will never go away.

---

1. Adapted from a 2022 Google search of poems and sayings.

Because those we love don't go away; they walk beside us every day, unseen, unheard, but always near, so loved, so missed, so very dear.

INTRODUCTION: HISTORICAL REFERENCES 01

Overview

The story of my sister's life is, in part, my life story, and because of this, I include several significant events, connections, and explanations that are the backdrop to the rest of the book. References to running; the onset of Betsy's illness; her first hospitalization; the genetic, environmental, and psychological connections; and why I did not have children will resonate with you.

Biographical information about my parents and insights regarding their personality are also included because for all Betsy's life, and particularly after she was diagnosed with bipolar disorder, they were her primary caregivers. Also, even though they did not see her again after 2001, they were in touch with her via telephone. I have written more about my father because his relationship with Betsy greatly impacted her life. This is discussed many times throughout this book.

Most of this book addresses a forty-year period—which is why some of the dates are not included—but the book is written in a quite accurate chronological order of what happened during Betsy's life.

Running for My Life

One of the ways that I coped with my sister's mental illness and the stress of daily life was by running. I ran for my physical and mental health and because I enjoyed it; my dear husband, Frank, was a long-distance runner and trained me to participate in my first marathon. Running cleaned out the cobwebs from my mind and provided an emotional outlet. Of course, it also kept me physically fit and, I believe, slowed down the aging process. I spent many hours running with Frank, alone, or with other runners, during which time I often thought about my sister and her life.

Throughout her life Betsy tried her best to exercise several times a day. She knew about my obsessive running and used to laugh about how much pain my husband and I experienced after finishing a long run. When Betsy and I were young, we participated in high school sports together—for example, the country club or high school swim team, as well as tennis and gymnastics. However, she was always faster and better at swimming and tennis than I was and tried out for the gymnastics team and was selected.

After 9/11, I remember reading about how the survivors at Cantor Fitzgerald, the investment banking firm, coped with the loss of most of their employees. They focused on rebuilding the company and donating money to the victims' families. During the many years of her illness, instead of being distracted by my concerns about Betsy, I immersed myself in the work I loved, which was one way I coped with her illness. (Passion is not a drug; it is a feeling.)

Overall, for over thirty years, running was a wonderful outlet that served many positive purposes. Without running, I believe I might have suffered a nervous breakdown. For example, there were days in the past when my sister caused me great distress, sadness, or anxiety, which in turn resulted in a major upheaval. A major upheaval could include crying, hang-up calls, and raised voices. Many times, with tears running down my face, I would put on my running shoes and clothes and dash out the door. After jogging for a few miles, I would feel the sweat run down my face, wait for the endorphins to kick in, and would feel better.

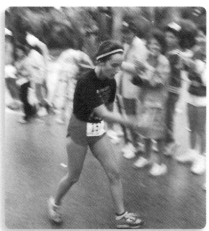

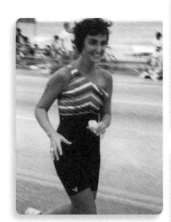

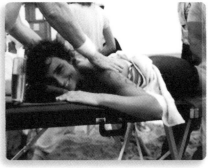

When you run you are not only relaxing your body, but you are also, in a sense, relaxing your mind. When this happens, you are more apt to open up to others and discuss problems of life.

In 1988 I participated in my second NYC Marathon with my dear husband Frank. The long run helped me to mentally deal with one of Betsy's horrible situations. She was incarcerated for six months for hitting a police officer, which was one of the many crises for which there was no end in sight. The finish line gave me an achievable ending. Thinking about the pain I was enduring during the last six miles of the marathon kept my tears away.

My father was going to give me a $500 savings bond if I completed the race in four hours or less. I missed it by sixteen minutes, but he gave me the bond anyway. I truly ran the marathon for my sister. Imagine this: running 26.2 miles, struggling to finish after an enduring side stitch for ten miles, while you know your sibling is locked up in jail for a crime committed when she was out of control and not responsible for her actions! What an unpleasant thought, but as I said earlier, this particular situation was not one of the worst. The number of miles I was running dictated how much discussion there was with my running partner, but there would always be bantering back and forth. Just the conversation reduced stress.

Writing Down My Stored Memories

During this time, I eventually came to realize that hiding in the closet, not speaking about my sister for fear of social rejection and judgment by peers and other people who don't understand mental illness, was not the answer. The battle was not only coping with and attempting to understand my sister's illness but also fighting my own internal battles and feelings about societal taboos. Although Betsy's illness interfered with her ability to acquire a job and hold a job (after 1989), causing her to become a noncontributing member of society and a ward of the state, her life did matter. The lives of disabled persons who suffer from horrific mental illnesses for which there are no known cures should be honored and remembered.

Eventually, I concluded that instead of storing my recollections concerning my sister's bipolar disorder in long term memory, they had to be written down. I decided I had to tell Betsy's story not only to justify my sister's life and my integral involvement with it, but also to share it to create a better understanding of mental illness. Anyone, any family, who has been drawn into a codependent relationship and has had to struggle to overcome suffering resulting from the destructive behavior patterns exhibited by a loved one, will want to read this book. Writing and completing this book has been a mentally and emotionally healing experience. It is also a way to remember my sister and to ensure that she will never be forgotten. I believe that sharing many intimate details of my life experience with my mentally ill sister will be interesting, sad, helpful, and beneficial to thousands of people.

Please note the following:

- In 2020, among the 52.9 million adults with any mental illness (AMI), 24.3 million (46.2%) received mental health services in the past year.

- More females with AMI (51.2%) received mental health services than males with AMI (37.4%).
- The percentage of young adults aged 18-25 years with AMI who received mental health services (42.1%) was lower than adults with AMI aged 26-49 years (46.6%) and aged 50 and older (48.0%).[2]

A recent NPR report on mental health and homelessness noted that "people with schizophrenia, for example, have died of hypothermia on the city's streets." Additionally, it cited Teresa Pasquini, an activist with NAMI whose son has schizophrenia, as saying that "the status quo has forced too many of our loved ones to die with their rights on" and for the last twenty years her son was "failed, jailed, treated, and streeted," by a broken public health system.[3]

I hope that when you finish reading this book, you may seek help for yourself, or if you have a family member or close friend who is mentally ill, you encourage them to seek some help and guidance. I implore you to be more accepting and understanding of mental illness in your family. As noted earlier, there are thousands of dysfunctional families in the United States whose dysfunctions are often directly related to their mentally ill family

2. "Mental Illness," National Institute of Mental Health (NIMH), 2020, https://www.nimh.nih.gov/health/statistics/mental-illness#part_2541.

3. April Dembosky, Amelia Templeton, and Carrie Feibel, "When Homelessness and Mental Illness Overlap, Is Forced Treatment Compassionate?" NPR, March 31, 2023, https://www.npr.org/sections/health-shots/2023/03/31/1164281917/when-homelessness-and-mental-illness-over-lap-is-compulsory-treatment-compassiona.

members. I was from a dysfunctional family (as of my sister's death, I am the only living member of my family on my father's side), but I survived. This book is a memoir about my life with my sister Betsy's bipolar disorder. I have compared my life with my sister to a rope with three sections—me, Betsy, and Betsy and me—wherein the rope would unravel, intertwine, tangle, tighten, or loosen, but never break, because I was always there for Betsy.

Events Leading Up to the Illness

The onset of Betsy's illness and everything that followed was never absent from my mind, and the most significant events set the stage for the rest of Betsy's life and mine.

It was during Betsy's last two years in high school (1970 to 1972) and first year in college that her illness emerged. As you can see by her pictures, she was beautiful then. Despite her beauty, her behavior was socially awkward and unusual. For example, she used to bring tons of schoolbooks to the beach. While everyone else drank beer and socialized, she read her schoolbooks and spent time thinking. She'd also bring her make-up and many changes of clothes with her. Why does someone need so many changes of clothes while sitting on the beach? Also, she was quite frequently stoned on marijuana or hash. When she was stoned, she had dilated eyes and loopy behavior while dressing, undressing, or reading and organizing books.

Sometime before Betsy graduated from high school (in 1972) in Dartmouth, Massachusetts, and before she was hospitalized (in 1975), one of the worst events in her life occurred. She was arrested for shoplifting; my father took action to keep it out of the newspaper. She knew wrong from right, was excelling in school, and was not needy, yet she was shoplifting in broad daylight and got caught. Why? Because she was compulsive and could not control her actions. Looking back over her entire life, I recall that she shoplifted on three occasions and was arrested twice. Her comment to me about one incident was, "They can't do anything to me; I'm a mental health case. It will get dismissed." It is interesting that after she finally accepted that she was bipolar, she used it as an excuse for aberrant behavior. My mother noticed this more than I did. Betsy was unable to delay gratification and did not seem to care about the consequences of her actions. I am not saying she had no remorse, guilt, or shame, but she did not apologize after the events that I knew about and discussed with her. In fact, each time she denied that she had shoplifted. Overall, Betsy did not seem to learn from her mistakes, and her compulsive behavior got her into trouble when it came to wanting an item she could not afford.

Even though she was stoned at times and had been arrested for shoplifting, she still excelled in school. The letter on the next page, dated February 20, 1974, is to Betsy from the dean of the College of Arts and Sciences at Southeastern Massachusetts University in North Dartmouth, Massachusetts (we lived in this town).

October 18, 1975, was when family life really changed. That date still, almost fifty years later, hangs on my heart. Betsy was diagnosed with a disorder. She had exhibited bizarre behavior prior to that October day, but my parents' assumptions were that it was due to drug usage. In fact, she was admitted to Butler Hospital at Brown University in Providence, Rhode Island, because of an overdose of quaaludes.

The Commonwealth of Massachusetts

Southeastern Massachusetts University

North Dartmouth, Massachusetts 02747

Dean

College of Arts and Sciences

February 20, 1974

Ms. Betsy Craig
56 Eleanor Street
North Dartmouth, Mass.   02747

Dear Ms. Craig:

Mr. Paul Fistori, our Director of University Records, has informed me that your cumulative average for the Fall Semester of 1973 was 4.000   .

This enables me the pleasure of placing your name on the Dean's List of the College of Arts and Sciences for this academic period.

My congratulations to you and I wish you continued success in your educational endeavors here at SMU.

Sincerely,

Joseph P. Sauro, Dean
College of Arts and Sciences

JPS:ps

cc: Mr. Paul Fistori
    Director of University Records

Shortly after that day, Mom and Dad came to visit me at my college for a long weekend. It was their twenty-fifth wedding anniversary and twenty-five years since Dad had graduated from college. A football game and many other festivities were scheduled on that cool autumn day in New Hampshire. The way I found out that Betsy was in the hospital was very shocking and very disturbing. Breaking the news to me was not what they expected to be the first part of their weekend. It came as a shock to me.

Sitting on the corner of my bed, Dad looked down and there was a long pause. "Your sister had a drug overdose and was admitted to Butler Hospital at Brown University. She'll be there for a while. We don't know what's wrong, but as you know, her behavior has been bizarre; she overdosed on some downers and has unusual mood changes." My mouth dropped. I was only eighteen, was dealing with my own issues in school and life, and was very upset when I heard the horrible news. I knew she had used drugs (marijuana, hashish), and so had I. The difference was I never abused any other drugs or overdosed. This was the first time I cried for Betsy. I did not realize then that the unexplained crying spells and overachieving behavior on my part and my sister's mental illness would drag into 2022. I also could not predict at that time that her illness would affect me my entire life, up until my sixties.

The weekend came to a close, and as Mom and Dad departed, I watched their car drive away. Feeling guilty, I thought that I was so lucky to be away at a private college in the mountains of New Hampshire when my sister was locked up in a psychiatric hospital. What could this be, and what would happen to her? My assumption was that the crisis would end soon. How naive we are when we are young, until we come to understand more about life and, in particular, the crippling effect mental illness has on you and your loved ones.

Now back to that fateful day in 1975. As soon as I left New

Hampshire and returned to Massachusetts, I went with Mom and Dad to visit my sister. She had been in group therapy and presented us with some crafts she made. Each one was very well done. She was really disoriented and apparently heavily medicated and almost appeared to be a zombie. I didn't understand, but I suspected that it was just due to drug abuse. Her diagnosis was as a manic-depressive. That was what my parents recalled the doctors called her illness in 1975. She was administered lithium and other medications. I didn't ask or desire to know what the drugs or medications could do and wouldn't have understood anyway. Earlier, I had completed a college course in abnormal psychology and read briefly about the disorder. All I remembered about it was that it was characterized by periods of mental highs and lows. Little did I or my parents know that 1975 was the beginning of a long, incurable illness that nearly destroyed their retirement years. Without my support and involvement, Betsy's illness might have bankrupted them. Little did we know then or ever anticipate that over thirty years later, she would become dependent on the very medications that were prescribed to stabilize her.

More about the First Hospitalization

Although Betsy's first hospitalization was discussed previously, I include additional information about it because of the way I remembered what she looked like and had going for her before the terrible date.

Betsy's hospitalization was the end of her life of normalcy, happiness, clarity, and accomplishable goal setting. But for us, the beginning was the start of a tragic downward spiral of a person who was one of the brightest, most beautiful, and most capable individuals, and who could have "had it all." I included several pictures of Betsy when she was in her twenties and thirties. She was very attractive and had beautiful hair, a great smile, an admirable figure, and a glow about her. The man in the picture was her long-term boyfriend, Scott, whose parents owned a liquor store (the picture is on the next page) in New Jersey. Some evenings he would work there, and she would accompany him. He wanted to marry her, but she declined. Over the years I have thought about him and wondered whether if she had married him, her life would have been better, because based on my experiences with him and how much he loved her, he would have probably taken very good care of her.

In the photos, her smiling face, engagement, and desire to pose for a picture indicate that she was stable on her medication. The pictures have given me a great deal of peace, knowing that at least some days of her life were happy and fulfilling. A picture tells a thousand tales.

Last Family Vacation

As if to compensate for her stay in an expensive private hospital and to mend a broken and distraught family, Dad made plans to take the family to Bermuda for a Christmas vacation. We were on the airplane leaving Boston during a terrible blizzard, and I thought we'd never get off the ground. Overall, the vacation was a total failure, not family oriented, and was unfortunately the last vacation we'd all spend together. Perhaps this is typical of some American families, but it may be an indication of a dysfunctional family. It isn't fun admitting this, either. Why were the vacation in 1975 and all other family holidays following that trip to Bermuda so upsetting and unpleasant? It was obviously my sister's behavior due to her bipolar disorder.

I believe it would have been different if not for my sister's illness. Alienation from and rejection of loved ones are among the many characteristics of bipolar disorder. Constant alienation and rejection are situations you must learn to cope with, although it often takes many years for some family members to be able to cope in a rational, nonemotional manner. Although I

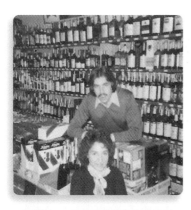
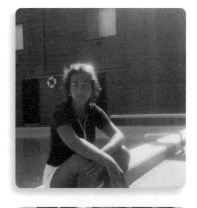
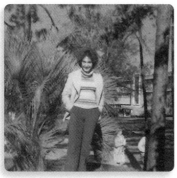
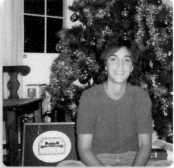

tried to enjoy myself in Bermuda, my sister generally had little or nothing to do with us. I wanted to spend some time with her, but she made it clear that she did not like being around me. Also, she either picked a fight with my father, my mother, or me (because she didn't like the way my father was reacting to her), or she was extremely sick and was unable to appropriately communicate.

During our trip to Bermuda in 1975, she always had some guy around. She not only ignored me but also spent most of the vacation with him. She even had the nerve to eat dinner in the dining room with him for a few nights instead of sitting with us. Whenever she spent time with us, she complained and then stayed as far away from us as she could.

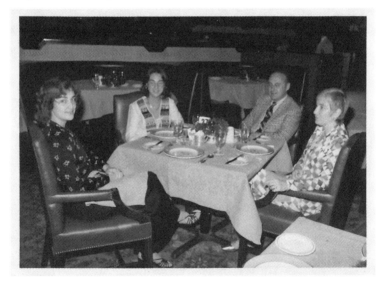

My mother kept a family photo of the four of us in the dining room at a resort in Bermuda for years. She kept it on her dresser. It is the only picture of our family together that my mother kept as a memory and hope that Betsy's life would be better.

At times I thought, "How ironic it is that one of the few holiday photos with all of us together is the one taken after my sister had gotten out of the psychiatric hospital in Providence, Rhode Island?"

Many Other Holidays

During many other Christmas holidays, years later, she spent a good part of the day calling us before going to my parents' home in Ormond Beach, Florida, and causing dissension (or attempting to). One Christmas, she couldn't decide when she would feel well enough to call us or arrive as planned, and used her need to sleep as an excuse. We wanted to wait as long as possible to open the gifts, so we would be together. However, we eventually jointly decided to open the gifts, as we felt strongly that her illness and mood shouldn't dictate our Christmas, as it had so many times before. We decided to let her open her gifts later in the day, after she arrived and before we ate our Christmas dinner.

The phone rang, and a man asked to speak to me; he was one of her new neighbors. He indicated that he could not give her a ride to my parents', and his inference was that no one was willing to pick her up. I was shocked. I didn't know the man and assured him that she would have transportation and would not spend the day alone. My mother and I went to pick her up. What my sister was doing was trying to set up a confrontation or gain sympathy from a neighbor. I call this behavior "histrionics," and I know that some of it was related to her erratic behavior, her need for attention, and her attempt to manipulate everyone.

The time she did spend with us was stressful, harried, upsetting, and worrisome. She opened her gifts, barely said "Thank you," and ate little of her dinner. Yet, as usual, she managed to fill her plate up with enough food for two people. After dinner she became agitated because my father would not accept a collect call from her estranged husband, who had previously beaten her up, wrecked her car, and caused much damage to her apartment. She couldn't understand why my father would not accept a collect call from a man who was also mentally ill, who had treated her so badly, and had abandoned her when she needed him. Instead of exhibiting rational behavior and understanding why my parents should not have to pay for his collect calls, she became agitated and started to lash out at everyone.

My other Christmas and Thanksgiving holidays were generally spent with some conflict. Holidays are exceedingly tough times when you have a mentally ill person in the family. With bipolar individuals, you never know what mood they will be in, whether or not they will be focused enough to eat when everyone else is eating, or whether they will cause some sort of emotional upheaval, which, of course, is always blamed on someone else. You come to expect a stressful time because the mentally ill person is not feeling quite right that particular day. We often felt that the behavior was for attention. However, attention getting is only one of the many tormenting and repetitive characteristics of the illness.

More about Betsy's Damaging Behaviors

Over the years there were many more painful, distressful, and heartbreaking times. On each occasion, I learned more about what was causing some of my negative thought processes and feelings of low self-esteem. Most of the feelings were a result of my sister's illness, which was a constant struggle. Throughout my early teens, my sister's emotionally damaging behaviors (before her official medical diagnosis and ongoing illness) consistently reared their ugly heads. At times I felt as though I was being punched and bitten by a five-headed serpent. And Betsy always implied that I caused the unpleasant incident. Her struggles were my struggles, and her behaviors toward me felt as if they were punches to my gut and psyche. I continually asked myself, "Why me? What did I do?" These questions did not help the quest I was on to build my self-esteem.

I finally came to understand that my sister could not control or eliminate her terrible moods. On the other hand, her thoughts sometimes were hopeful and uplifting. Several of the most noteworthy letters and cards appear throughout the book. I tried to put myself in her shoes, as difficult as it was. She was often not only lonely but had great difficulty dealing with her mood swings and the gain and then loss of friends. She was smart enough to identify her moods. Regardless, she attended a family event anyway, and when everyone else was acting normal and she was not, she became paranoid and lashed out. Still, I tried to put myself in her shoes and remain calm and understanding. However, this selfless act exhausted me more times than I can count.

I can't begin to verbalize and put in writing how many times she made a fiasco out of it—for example, storming out before dinner, chugging champagne when she knew she shouldn't drink while on medication, and then getting angry when reminded that drinking while on medications could result in adverse effects. Her name-calling and other verbal abuse was also very common.

Part of her unhappiness was due to what my parents were not able to provide for her. For example, they would not pay for her to live on the campus of Brown University in Providence, Rhode Island, because we lived twenty-five minutes from the campus, and she would have preferred to have a new car instead of the use of a VW Beetle our father bought for her. I strongly surmise that her anger was caused by what I call the traumatic or haunting side of the disorder. When your inner self feels so negative to the point of contemplating suicide (my sister attempted this on a few occasions and threatened it frequently), it is hard to be positive about the rest of your life. However, it was also difficult to determine which of her stories and comments about wanting to kill herself were fabrications and which were not, particularly when they were attention-getting tactics.

When bipolar individuals are in crisis, no matter how small or trivial the situation may seem to a normal person, everyone is lured in. If you are codependent, as my parents and I were, you are going to get dragged down and worn out by their frantic cries for help. A tactic I used besides putting myself in her shoes was to repeat to myself how horrific and sad her life was and that I should be there for her and appreciate what I had.

As I continued to deal with my sister's difficulties, the way she verbally abused me and my parents and displayed other lashing-out behavior, I would get caught up in ruminating about what I had to endure and often forgot to consider what she had to endure. Moreover, being a parent, sibling, or close relative of someone with a brain disease affects everyone in unusual ways. But as a strong survivor of the chaotic ups and downs of dealing with a mentally ill family member, I learned that it was how I dealt with my sister's illnesses and my own codependency that counted. Strategies for coping are referenced in each chapter but are the major theme of The Stages of Healing chapter of this book.

Some Findings about the State of Health Care

Many of the findings of the "State of Mental Health Care in America" report (2023) are relevant to my sister's life:

- In 2019–2020, 20.78% of adults were experiencing a mental illness. That is equivalent to over 50 million Americans.
- Millions of adults in the United States experience serious thoughts of suicide, with the highest rate among multiracial individuals. The percentage of adults reporting serious thoughts of suicide is 4.84%, totaling over 12.1 million individuals. In 2020 serious thoughts of suicide were reported by 11% of adults who identified with two or more races–6% higher than the average among all adults.
- More than 1 in 10 youth in the United States are experiencing depression that is severely impairing their ability to function at school or work, at home,

with family, or in their social life. Suffering from at least one major depressive episode (MDE) in the past year is reported by 16.39% of youth (age 12-17), and 11.5% of youth (over 2.7 million youth) are experiencing severe major depression.

- Nationally, 1 in 10 youth who are covered under private insurance do not have coverage for mental or emotional difficulties—totaling over 1.2 million youth. In Arkansas (ranked 51), nearly one-quarter of youth with private insurance do not have coverage for mental health care.[4]

If my father did not have excellent health insurance when my sister was diagnosed with bipolar disorder in 1975, she would have never been admitted to Butler Hospital at Brown University for treatment. And because my mother was very intelligent, a voracious reader, and had excellent administrative skills, she was finally able in 1989 to get my sister on Social Security Disability Insurance benefits. Fortunately, my sister had enough of a work history to be awarded some benefits. Had she not had the benefits when she lived in Florida and when she moved to New Jersey and then New York, she would never have received any treatment. She could have ended up on the streets.

Genetic, Environmental, and

4. Maddy Reinert, Theresa Nguyen, and Danielle Fritze, "The State of Mental Health in America 2023," Mental Health America, October 2022, https://mhanational.org/sites/default/files/2023-State-of-Mental-Health-in-America-Report.pdf.

Psychological Connections

Serious mental illnesses are brain diseases, biologically based, and are no one's "fault." As with physical illness, there are many distinct kinds of mental illness, with many different causes. Mental illnesses are *not* the result of weak character or bad parenting.[5]

- In 2020, among the 52.9 million adults with AMI, 24.3 million (46.2%) received mental health services in the past year.
- More females with AMI (51.2%) received mental health services than males with AMI (37.4%).
- The percentage of young adults aged 18-25 years with NAMI who received mental health services (42.1%) was lower than adults with AMI aged 26-49 years (46.6%) and aged 50 and older (48.0%).[6]
- And in the first year of the COVID-19 pandemic, global prevalence of anxiety and depression increased by a massive 25%, according to a scientific brief released by the World Health Organization (WHO).[7]

---

5. NAMI brochure, 1993.

6. National Institute of Mental Health. "Mental Illness," National Institute of Mental Health (website), last updated March 2023. https://www.nimh.nih.gov/health/statistics/mental-illness.

7. Nirmita Panchal, Heather Saunders, Robin Rudowitz, and Cynthia Cox, "The Implications of COVID-19 for Mental Health and Substance Use," KFF, March 20, 2023, https://www.kff.org/coronavirus-covid-19/issue-brief/the-implications-of-covid-19-for-mental-health-and-substance-use/.

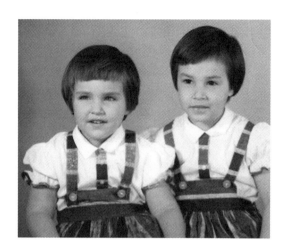

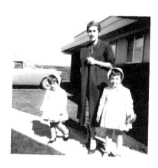

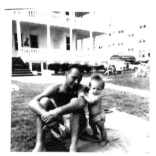

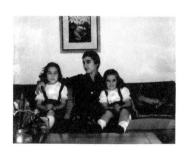

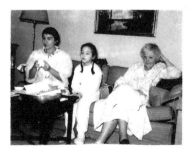

Linsey Willis

My Great-Grandmother Sue Abbott Throop

My great-grandmother Sue Abbott Throop, who was born October 17, 1870, in Cincinnati, Ohio, was bipolar. Below is a picture of Sue Abbott Throop at eight years of age, taken on September 25, 1878. My mother and father told me that Sue was never diagnosed with a disorder.

My parents believed that there was a genetic link between Sue Throop, my paternal great-grandmother, and my sister because of what my dad recalled about her behavior when he was growing up. Because Sue lived with my father's parents later in her life, he interacted with her a great deal. Dad's parents never provided him with any definitive proof of this, but he surmised it based on his observations of Sue.

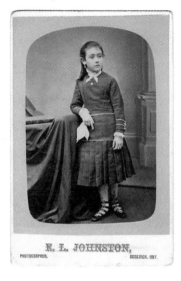

E. L. JOHNSTON,
PHOTOGRAPHER,   GODERICH, ONT.

A discussion about a genetic link is included because I believe it helps to better understand and explain Betsy's behavior. Also, because my father recalled what Sue Throop was like while he was dealing with Betsy's illness, he told me and my mother that he slowly, and reluctantly, accepted that my sister was not to blame for her mental illness. Additionally, I include information about my father's personality (later in this section) because, based on my life experience dealing with him and his attitude and behavior toward Betsy, I believe it exacerbated her illness.

In other words, she had difficulty dealing with his sometimes dogmatic, controlling, critical, and oftentimes distant and uncaring behaviors.

IN MEMORIAM

GEORGE HUNTINGDON THROOP

Lieut.-Colonel, 24th Engineers, A.E.F., U.S.A., 1917 - 1919

Similar to Betsy's behavior, Sue's behavior, as my dad recalled, was also bizarre. My father had difficulty recalling and articulating specifics about the behaviors. He did recall some positive traits; Sue was a good poet and published a book of poetry. Sadly, my aunt threw it out after her parents passed away. What an unfortunate decision. The following is one of the poems which my father had saved.

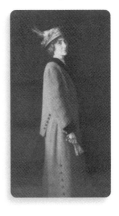

Like Betsy, Sue was highly creative and did artwork and painted. My sister's greatest gifts were her brilliant mind, writing ability, creativity, and sense of humor.

My great-grandmother was known for leaving home and being gone for many days, while no one knew where she was. Also, during the last years of her life, my grandfather totally supported her.

A SOLDIER PASSES

So green and cool among the sunny stones
        the grasses 'round him creep;
So tenderly the sky bends down
        in her blue cloak to wrap him!
Over the quiet breast the noble banner's folds
Majestic lie.
        The wind is still . . .

        . . . "Forasmuch as it hath pleased
Almighty God to take our comrade . . . Who labored
not in vain . . . faithful to duty . . . unto death . . . "

        . . . To duty . . .
Unto death . . . Under this sky from whose deep bosom
So many mercies flow—how shall war's savageries
Be duty? Still shall dark ages call on men to die
For these? . . .

        No! Not for these; but what transcends them.
War is more than swords and shrapnel on a bloody field;
More than our reasons why.
        For every greater light
A Calvary! The world is built
Of hero-gifts strewing blind trails
Whereon men see but darkly; yet with broken feet
And faces lit, gloriously seek for Truth . . .

Out of the dubious shadows of those trails
Our Fathers, single-minded, caught Promethean fire
To weld pure gold into our corner-stone.
        The banded clouds,
The stars studding the fathomless empyrean
They chose for blazon; under which should go
Forever,—guarding our birthright, carrying on,—
Legions with proud, uplifted foreheads . . .
        Never
Changeling, slavish mobs whining to Life
To pamper them!

        . . . Oh God—preserve our Nation's head
Unbowed!

        . . . Solemn the Chaplain's words and friendly
Fall—"Our parting tribute . . . "
        So!—the last salute . . .
See how it wreathes a nimbus over him!
Taps! . . .
        Time to leave him to his sleep . . .

Anne Throop Craig
New York. August 11, 1938.
Reprinted from "St. Thomas's Weekly", Mamaroneck, N. Y.

I don't know if she was ever hospitalized, but she was lucky to not have been sent to a mental institution. Sadly, more than one hundred years ago, people like her were sent to state mental hospitals, often called *insane asylums,* which they more than likely never left and very rarely saw their relatives.

Some of you may recall the story about one of the daughters of Joseph P. Kennedy and his wife Rose. Their daughter's behavior and actions became uncontrollable, and a harsh decision was made to give her a lobotomy, which, according to what I read, was to save his career. In her early young-adult years, Rosemary Kennedy experienced seizures and violent mood swings. In response to these issues, her father arranged a prefrontal lobotomy for her in 1941, when she was twenty-three years of age; the procedure left her permanently incapacitated and rendered her unable to speak intelligibly.[8] Additionally, "Rosemary Kennedy would spend the rest of her life institutionalized and isolated from her family."[9]

Even though my descriptions of my father's personality are not positive, he had many very good qualities, and over the years, at times, he was nice, fun, and easy to be around. I did love him but sometimes wondered if he loved me. For example, he took me to golf tournaments with him, and I would ride in the golf cart. He also taught me about golfing. Sometimes he helped me with one of my favorite chores, which was raking and picking up leaves. He would also often take my mom, sister, and me to dinner at very nice restaurants and the country club, and when I was an adult, we often spent many hours playing backgammon.

I never knew anything about my great-grandfather or much more than what I previously describe about my great-grandmother, Sue, and was grateful to learn something when my father finally shared the information.

---

8. "Rosemary Kennedy," Wikimedia Foundation, last modified May 6, 2023, 21:25 (UTC), https://en.wikipedia.org/wiki/Rosemary_Kennedy.

9. Kate Serena, "The Forgotten Story of Rosemary Kennedy, Who Was Lobotomized So That JFK Could Succeed," All That's Interesting, last updated May 2, 2022, https://allthatsinteresting.com/rosemary-kennedy.

When my sister's illness commenced, my parents were united in their initial efforts to save her, and I followed their lead. However, I have no idea the extent to which my grandparents tried to save Sue Throop, which is particularly relevant, given that she was born in 1870.

The family needs to be united when dealing with a loved one with mental illness. We learned this over many difficult and trying years. Being united should also involve spending time learning about yourselves through individual, group, or family therapy, which is important because you might be able to prevent tragic consequences such as a drug overdose, suicide attempt, or suicide.

My dad's sister, Mary Ann, kept many of her parents' papers when they passed away, and then she gave them to my parents. After my parents passed away, I read the papers and then locked them in our safe. I decided to review the papers to see if there was anything more I could learn about my family background and particularly about my great-grandmother.

I found what I feel is a fairly well-written, flowery, and interesting letter my great-grandmother Sue wrote to my grandfather when he was a young man. I learned some interesting things about England. My grandfather wanted to know more about his ancestors. Based on the color of the paper and the fact that it is very fragile, I estimate it to be about one hundred years old. What a treasure.

For. Robert Throop Craig.

You asked me for some data, dear Bob, as to family
matters. Here is some ,and I will write more interesting
things when I have more time,soon.

I was born in Cincinnati in 1870,according to
mamma's notes on a baby photograph or so,- though on
others,1869,(October 17,)

Your grandmother,my mother, was Mary Jane Catherine
(Abbot) Throop and was born in Washington,D.C. in 1842.
She met my father, Everett Sheridan Throop,during the Civil War,
in Cincinnati, where she had gone to visit her aunt, Lucy(Abbot)
Kebler(Mrs. John Kebler). My father was in the war service at
that time, andon furlough, wounded. He had just n xxxxxxxxxx
been admitted to the Bar of Cincinnati, and begun to practice law
(he was twenty fouryears old) when the war broke out and he joined
the "Guthrie Grays" the crack,young men's regiment of the county.
My mother became engaged to him, and then had to go abroad with
her father, who was appointed to direct a consular district in
England.(He was George Jacob Abbot,and had been distinguished
as an educationalist in Washington, for he entirely reconstructed
the public school system there. The Abbot School in Washington,
is named for him.) He had been at the head of the Consular Bureau
in Washington during the Civil War.

My grandmother had died when mother was seventeen,so
the latter was head of my grandfather s house in Sheffield,Eng
land. ABout1867 mother came back to America and was married
in April,1868 to Everett S. Throop,in Portland,Maine, at my
great grandfather's house,there, a beautiful old place where we
used to visit great aunts,then living, when we were children,

and where we went when my father died,in 1881.) This house is
now torn down, the gardens and orchard sold and a Polish church
stands on the site.)

This great grandfather was on my grand maternal grandmother's
side, and was Nicholas Emery, who was Judge of the Supreme Court
of Maine. His portrait is that fine one which Auntie Lu Nichols
and Mother had in their drawing room in Cambridge, though it was
first willed to Aunt Annie Morison and hung in their dinding
room on Farrar Street in Cambridge. Judge Emery's wife was
a daughter of John Taylor Gilman, fourteen terms first Colonial
Governor of New Hampshire,and his portrait is that of the exceeding
ly plain gentleman in gown and queue in the dining room at
mother's,in Cambridge! But plain or not,-as he certainly was.-
he was said to have been a distinguished and as well, most
charming nd witty gentleman!

My mother's family were: myself,1869; Lucy Abbot Throop,
b. June,10,1871; Mary Susan Everett Throop, Dec 12,1872;
George William Huntingdon Throop,Nov.8,1875 (or 76); and
August 1878 (Or 79)
Everett Abbot Throop,1879: (Everett died in 1895,September,after
one year at Harvard,where he should never have gone so young
and not strong, growing too fast; and never would have gone till
another year, if mamma had followed her own best judgment and
other people who knew too much hadn't pooh-poohed her out of it!
It was unintelligent and stupid; he was a most lovely boy,with
a beautiful singing voice and a fine mind.)
Nov. 1867   C. J. S.
Your father was born in Germany. His life was happy
at first, them after his mother died his father married an inferior,
ambitious woman, and from that time the life of the two children,
(boys) was uncertain and at length tragic. I will tell about it
in another letter.

My father's family has a very romantic background; my mother's a rather particularly scholarly and quieter ancestry.

My father's ancestor in this country, the first one, was William Throop (originally Scrope) The change of name is interesting in its cause. I don't know whether I have ever told you this story. Here it is:

William Scrope was the eldest son of Col. Adrien Scrope, one of the regicides who brought about the execution of Charles 1st. When the Stuarts were reinstated on the throne, after Cromwell's regime had passed, Adrien Scrope with other regicides, was impri soned, then executed, and the estates of his heirs confiscated by the Crown. His eldest son fled to Scotland, and later became embroiled in some Scottish rebellion, and fled to America. That was in 1637 (or 1647). He settled in Rhode Island, first, then went to Connecticutt, near where Hartfor d now is, a place called Lebanon. A number of other young regicides' sons were there also, so that their community was known as "The Regicides."

This William, because the Scrope line was now in ill favor with the English Crown, and because the his new home was still colonial, for safety, took a name of his mother's family, Throop. (His mother was a daughter of a Lord Clifford , a Scottish peer.) William had seberal children, among them a Benjamin, and a Daniel. Daniel was my father's direct ancestor, four generations back from my father's father. This Daniel's descendants, one of them went to New York state, and settled in what is now Madison County, and my, father was born in Hamilton, there. His mother was *Calpurnia* *(Sanders)* Dunbar. The descendants of the Benjamin Throops, went to New York state, also, but settled in Ontario County, which is where I visited some of the family last summer. (I will tell you more about this, later. It is romantic and interesting.)

The history of the Scrope family is interesting,also, before the descendants came to this c untry.

The first Scrope in England was a Norman by descent,and was made First Baron Scrope in 1397 by Richard (II,I think) or IV? He was a very powerful lord, for he was made ruler of the Isle of Mann, Warden of the West Marshes (which I think is about the Northumberland region) and had granted him by Richard, the whole demesne of Wiltshire. The Scrope peerage is the oldest in England and was for a number of generations themost powerful,was so, anyway until according to history, the 11th baron kicked up,and behaved badly, by having a large number of illegitimate sons whose mothers were powerful ladies of rank, so that when he died without legit imate issue, these other heirs all fell upon his estates, thus dividing and greatly minimizing them. From that time thepower of this peerage appears to have declined.

after Baron Scrope, the First, my father's direct line But ~~thazfterkzBaronxScrapezwaszaaxzkhazdireakxanonsxoxxafx~~ ~~nyxfatherzxikzwawzhinzkhirdzbratkerzxStephenx waaxthexthirdxnoma~~ ~~xan~~ was from the third son, Stephen Scrope,was who was Earl of something or other,-(Cockerington, perhaps,though I forget the record here.) This line of course was never so powerful as the that which was issue of the eldest brother of the First Baron's sons; also, these younger brother's (two) lines appear to have been more god-fearing, and at the same time, much more radical and democratic, Stephen's descendant, a drious, anyway,- for they threw in their allegiance with the Commonwealth of Cromwells regime, and fought on that side for the people against the luxurious and weak Stuart kings(Which I'm glad to know of them. For this more manly stand ,of course,they lost their estates, when Adrien was beheaded; but in a good cause! They were brave and independent men; and the Throope have been so in this country since;about which I th tell you,as I say, in another letter ?......

Robert Throop Craig

My paternal grandfather, Robert Throop Craig, was an interesting, intelligent, thoughtful, but eccentric man. You can't tell by the picture when he was in his early sixties. Also, he saved the newspaper article about himself.

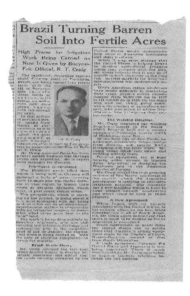

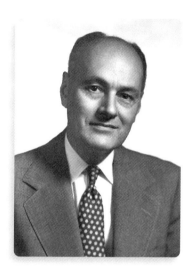

For his entire career, Robert Throop Craig worked for a multinational corporation, Ruston Bucyrus, Ltd. He was the senior vice president of marketing. He and my grandmother Helen lived in Milwaukee, Wisconsin, in a mansion and employed a full-time butler and maid.

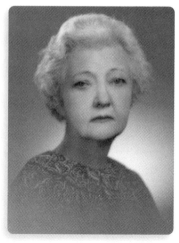

Every evening he required my father to wear a jacket to dinner. My father kept it in a downstairs closet. Although he was never diagnosed or treated, based on my knowledge, my paternal grandfather was an obsessive-compulsive personality. For example (and he showed me his logs), he kept track of every single mile he drove in his car, kept many handwritten lists and records of accounts, etcetera.

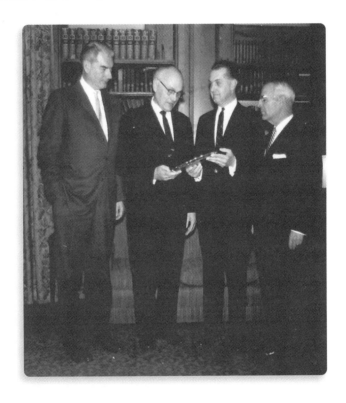

He not only kept many lists, but like my father, he also saved the lists. A very interesting part of a several-page-list follows. He kept track of all of his trips from 1931 to 1960.

R. T. CRAIG'S TRAVEL ABROAD - 1931 thru 1960

PASSPORT 352319 - Issued Washington 3/24/31
        Renewed   "   10/3/34
        Expired   "   3/24/35

1931

Entered France(Cherbourg)	. . . . .	April 14, 1931
Entered Switzerland(Vallorbe)	. . .	April 19, 1931
Entered Greece	. . . .	April 21, 1931
Left Greece	. . . .	August 7, 1931
Entered, England(Dover)	. . . . . .	August 11, 1931
Entered U.S.A.	. . . .	August 23, 1931

1932

Entered France(Cherbourg)	. . .	July 23, 1932
Entered Greece	. . . .	July 25, 1932
Left Greece	. . . .	August 9, 1932
Entered Italy(Brindisi)	. . . .	August 9, 1932
Entered France	. . . .	August 11, 1932
Entered England(Croydon)	. . . .	August 13, 1932
Entered U.S.A.	. . . .	August 26, 1932

1934

Entered France(Cherbourg)	. . .	October 11, 1934 (Vals de Loire)
Left France(LeHavre)	. . . . .	November 14, 1934
Entered England(Southampton)	. .	November 14, 1934
Entered France(Boulogne-sur-Mer)		November 21, 1934
Entered Czechoslovakia	. . . . .	November 22, 1934
Entered England(Dover)	. . . . .	December 11, 1934
Entered U.S.A.	. . . .	December 22, 1934

PASSPORT 181447 - Issued Washington 4/23/35

1936

Entered Chile(Arica)	. . . . . .	July 31, 1936
Entered U.S.A.	. . . .	September 22, 1936

1937/1947 (see under) (Page 1a)

PASSPORT 265085 - Issued Washington 8/19/48
              Renewed   8/1/51

1948

Entered Southampton	. . . .	9/28/48
Left Southampton	. . . .	10/14/48
Entered Stockholm, Sweden	. . .	10/14/48
Left Stockholm, Sweden	. . .	10/21/48
Entered Zurich, Switzerland	. .	10/21/48
Left Zurich, Switzerland	. . .	10/23/48
Entered Amsterdam, Holland	. . .	10/23/48
Left Amsterdam, Holland	. . .	10/24/48
Entered Brussels, Belgium	. . .	10/24/48
Left Brussels, Belgium	. . .	10/26/48

And as you observed from the list, he traveled frequently all over the world. My grandmother said he'd often be gone for a month or two at a time to Europe and would travel by ship. My mother did not favor him because she said he was anti-Semitic. She told me a story about when he returned to the United States on the Queen Mary. He made a comment, something to the effect of, "I am so glad I was on the upper deck. The Jews and peasants are in the lower decks or in the steerage section." When I asked him about it, he denied ever making that statement.

The fact that he was accused of being an anti-Semite had no impact on my life until I was in my early teens, when I found out that I had Jewish ancestry. I knew that both of my mother's parents were from Russia and arrived in the United States in 1917, at the height of the Bolshevik Revolution, but not that they were Jewish. However, what our parents tried to overcome impacts all of us greatly as children.

He would also repeat himself many times about the same subject in letters and in person, during the few times I spent with him during my adult life. Those are obsessive-compulsive behaviors. He was also the kind of man who had to keep up with the Joneses and never seemed to be content with his lifestyle. Perhaps he was trying to overcome what he had come from and just wanted more for his family. I believe wanting to keep up with the Joneses was important to some families who grew up during the Depression years.

Despite these examples of his oddities, he wrote me wonderful letters, and I wrote him back. It was a wonderful and lifelong pen pal relationship, and I learned a great deal about life when reading each of his letters.

My grandfather complained to me in the letters he wrote to me that that my father didn't pay enough attention to him and my grandmother. Apparently, my father knew that his father and mother had difficulty with the fact that we didn't visit often but did nothing about it except to see them when my father was on the West Coast on business. As noted previously, my grandfather was too miserly to spend the money to visit us after they retired to California. However, he had paid very little attention to my father when he was growing up, so what should my grandfather have expected? My father's behavior in respect to visiting Betsy and me was the same.

The following letter, which includes comments from my grandmother Helen on the sides and tops of the pages, is a bit difficult to read because of the beautiful handwriting. My grandfather commented on the lack of communication from my parents, my dad's short visit with them, my career, and the fact that he was pleased that I had broken up with a boyfriend, whom he referred to as a peasant. At the time the comment did not bother me, but if he were alive today and referred to someone as a peasant, I would advise him of my discomfort with it.

Dear Linsey - We do thank you for taking time
out of your busy day to write to us and we
are grateful. It was great of you to remember
us also write a pretty V- card.

ROBERT T. CRAIG
3426 A BAHIA BLANCA W
LAGUNA HILLS
CALIFORNIA 92653

Feb. 14, 1981

Dear Linsey,

Thank you for your
letter of Jan. 29th and for the
Valentine. We very much appreciate
your continuing effort to keep in
touch with us and are glad that
you rate us "special". This will
assure us, we hope, of at least some
contact with the Junior Craig family
which, alas, is not noteworthy in
the matter of communication.

I have noted the termination
of your affair with the Israeli peasant
and can't help wondering why you
fell for him in the first place, having
regard for his flaws of character which you
now have outlined to us. As to revival
of your friendship with two "old flames"
please look up the word "platonic"
in your dictionary. It may enable you
to understand why I am anxious to

know which one of them you prefer.

I am glad that you are again working in the warehouse, because you are happier there than you apparently were in the store — and because you seem to think you can remain there, content for a year and a half. I hope by then you will be able to decide on the basic elements essential to a degree of stability which you have not appeared to attain thus far. If I may make just one suggestion in this connection — concentrate on the job and put the boy friends in second place. You are young and have plenty of time for the latter and in the meantime you may be able to determine what qualities are more important as a basis for a lasting friendship.

Yes, your father came to see us and we had a few hours to enjoy with him — but on these business trips he is usually under pressure and so we seldom have time to cover all the things we'd like to talk about.

I looked forward to reading his letters and responded back to them. He was a highly intelligent man, and even though he indicated that he did not attend college, he was a very good writer.

My sister also wrote wonderful letters and sent beautiful cards to me her entire life. Writing was a family characteristic. Many of Betsy's letters are included in this book because the contents shed additional light on her thought processes and illness.

Many people spend most of their lives trying to overcome the family from which they came, particularly if one or more persons are afflicted with a mental illness. The family member's mental illness may be totally ignored, may be misunderstood, or excuses may be made about the illness instead of doing something to help the person. Over the years, I have met several people who mentioned that they had a mentally ill sibling or relative but had nothing to do with them. When I heard this, I was horrified.

As stated previously, my grandfather spent very little time with my father, and history repeated itself with my father. Both of them were out of town a great deal on business and then tended to their social interests (e.g., golfing, bridge, playing cards) when not working. Many of us repeat the behaviors and actions we grew up with, and therefore, the cycle is not broken. This is demoralizing because sometimes the cycle damages the family. I do not mean to imply that totally nurturing parents will prevent any type of mental illness from emerging. I believe it means that time spent with children helps to build better self-esteem and closeness. And therapy will help people recognize the behaviors and actions they are repeating.

My Father, Robert T. Craig, Jr.

My father grew up in Milwaukee, Wisconsin, and attended a prep school in the countryside. During his youth (1924 to 1950), he lived very well. After coming home from WWII, he attended and graduated from Brown University.

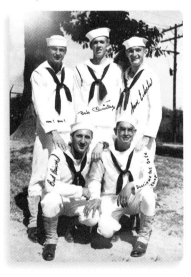

Given that most of our WWII veterans are deceased and many wonderful pictures have been lost, I include a picture of my father and his shipmates. He kept an original photo, autographed by men who served on the US Navy destroyer in WWII, as well as a picture of the ship, the USS *Madison*. My dad is the person at the top left.

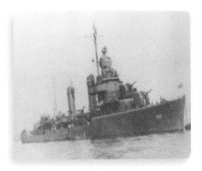

Do the pictures that follow give you any insight into the kind of life he lived and the person he was? He cared a great deal about his looks during his entire life. He was a great dresser and only wore designer brands (e.g., Brooks Brothers and Florsheim wingtip shoes). My father was a bit of a narcissist (he was never diagnosed for this, however), but then again, aren't many successful people? When my parents had parties, he always had to be the center of attention. He carefully controlled the opening of our Christmas gifts and made us clean up the paper immediately after opening each gift. I did not particularly like that he controlled the process, but he did this so everyone would take time to review each gift. He also demonstrated many obsessive behaviors which often hurt the ones he loved. Betsy could not stand that he had to be the center of attention, but she was the same way! Their similar personalities often clashed, which was destructive because they would get in an argument and one of them would tell the other to shut-up, given Betsy's illness.

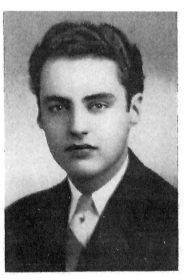

ROBERT CRAIG

Entered 9th Form; Glee Club 11; Rifle Club; Football 11, 12C; Basketball 10, 11, 12C; Baseball 9, 10C, 11C, 12C; Fitch Improvement Prize 10.

Bob's forte at Country Day has been athletics, and his achievements in this field are enviable. As center on the football team, Bob's fighting spirit was always present. This year he was starting forward on the basketball five, and has been a regular infielder in baseball. Outside of school his chief interest lies in his best friends. He has worked hard to acquire his grades and in return has won the Improvement Prize. It was indeed fortunate that Bob was permitted to finish the year at Country Day through the kindness of his draft board.

My father and grandfather demonstrated similar characteristics and behaviors. For example, my dad reminded me that he and my mother had to borrow $150 to get married, and his parents made an issue about attending the wedding because of travel costs, which they told him they could not afford. When my grandparents moved from California to Wisconsin after he retired in 1963, they never flew back East to visit us, and the reason was he said they could not afford to. He and my grandfather were obsessive about saving money and keeping track of all expenditures.

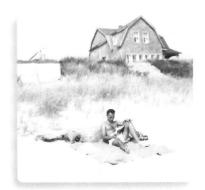
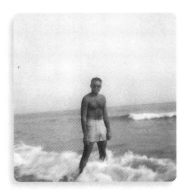
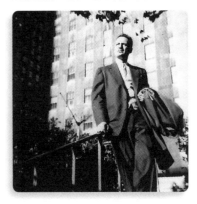
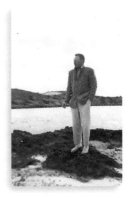

My parents were married in 1950. My father never forgot his experience of growing up in a mansion and then being told by his father that he had to pay for his wedding. I remember this well because he told me on many occasions that when he got married, he had a hole in his shoe, and although his parents attended the small ceremony, they did not give him a wedding present. When I got married at age thirty-three, and without asking him to pay for my wedding, he told me he could not afford to pay for it. Of course, he could have, but I told him I did not want him to pay for it, as my fiancé, Frank, and I could pay for it ourselves. Of course, I was a bit upset, but because I was conditioned to his behavior, I did not let it upset me. I just thought he did not want to spend the money. However, even though my father was not generous about some issues, he had no problem paying for his daughters' college and graduate school education.

Another example has to do with my great-grandmother. My father told me that his father had to take care of his grandmother, and once again history was repeated because my father also took care of my sister. Nonetheless, talking about the financial costs or burdens does not cure the illness or resolve the problems the illness causes. Genetic characteristics and illnesses including those not diagnosed by a professional, pass down through the generations.

My father had the habit of making fun of and criticizing his sister, and he did the same to me. During my last visit to see my grandparents, which was three months before my grandfather passed away, both of them were reminiscing and told me they were sorry that my father and his father had been so critical of his sister.

Unfortunately, because my father was not a touchy-feely person, he only occasionally hugged me or showed compassion, interest, or sympathy. Limited emotional support amplified the problems with my sister's illness. *Sympathy* is a key word here.

Body language is a powerful, significant, large, and meaningful part of communication, and my father's behavior told a story. At times he would have a big frown or would roll his eyes, or when he was speaking, he would use a tone of voice that made the person feel as though they were being talked down to. Sometimes when I cried, he showed no sympathy. On other occasions, his beautiful blue eyes, which I was lucky to inherit, appeared to be shedding tears. His eyes had a story to tell. His way of dealing with problems was to take the bull by the horns and solve them, no matter how offensive his actions came off to the recipient. He would say that he was pragmatic and that being emotional would not help resolve a difficult situation. Over the years I grew to appreciate his pragmatism.

However, deep down inside, over all the years of my sister's illness, my father was distraught about it, and sometimes he did shed a tear or two in front of my mother and me. Nevertheless, there were times when he should or could have demonstrated more concern for my sister's condition, and he remained stand-offish. Throughout Betsy's life, she craved his attention and sympathy but did not receive it very often. As I recall, much of the attention our father provided was in the form of criticism, directive, and teaching.

Being pragmatic and using sound judgment and logic are good strategies to employ, but to a mentally ill person, good judgment and logic are not part of their thought process. For example, when my sister had to have her entire set of teeth replaced, he paid for the process in two stages because this made better financial sense. I believe the process took three to six months. My dad would use certificates of deposit (CDs) that reached maturity to pay for extra expenses. To my sister it was cruel and unusual punishment. I agreed with her and, many times, viewed him as self-centered and a tightwad. Although he was frugal his entire life, as noted previously, he paid for all my and my sister's undergraduate and graduate educations. I will never forget this, and his generosity helped make me who I am today. Without the education, I would have never had a linear career.

While we were growing up, Betsy and I used to refer to my father as the Ogre, because he was so stern, dogmatic, distant, grumpy, and mean at times. He also had a tendency to talk down to us, not allowing us to interrupt him, and demanded full attention when he called a family meeting. We were to listen, and he was to talk and not be interrupted nor disagreed with. He also was not one to engage in small talk and would rather read a book or watch football, golf, or other sports than chitchat with us. He had difficulty engaging in what he referred to as wasted conversation. Throughout Betsy's life she referred to him as the Ogre, but her poor judgment, occasional paranoia, and inability to manage her finances were a few reasons why my father often had to behave like an ogre. I believe that because of his obsessive-compulsive behavior, he could not help how he acted. When I told him many years later that I thought he demonstrated obsessive-compulsive behavior and that I took after him, he laughed. After we finished watching the Oscar-Award-winning movie *As Good as It Gets*, with Jack Nicholson and Helen Hunt, and I told him that at times he acted like Jack Nicholson's character, he laughed and said he agreed with me.

When Jack Nicholson answered his door, he was rude to Cuba Gooding Jr., and my father was rude to some people when they rang our doorbell. Jack Nicholson ate at the same diner every morning at the same time and at the same table. He also ordered the exact same breakfast every morning and made sure the same waitress, Helen Hunt, served him every day. My father ate the same breakfast at the same time every morning and sat in the same chair. He was a creature of habit.

I never loathed my father and did love him but was sad that he was not more nurturing. My mother, Joan, who I loved a great deal, was very nurturing, which was a saving grace. Betsy either adored or loathed him and told him this, and I could see the sadness in his face and eyes. I believe her illness contributed to her difficulty in dealing with him, particularly because he was not nurturing. Later on in my life, I had a great deal of respect and admiration for my father because he helped make me who I became. As stated previously, not only did he pay for all my college and graduate education, but he also showed great concern or interest in the men I dated, took great care of my mother, and took great care of his estate planning such that when he passed on, all t's were crossed and i's dotted. My husband referred to it as a turnkey operation.

My Mother, Joan Renee Pickard

My mother, Joan, was born in Gloversville, New York, on March 6, 1927, and graduated from Pleasantville High School in Pleasantville, New York. She then graduated from Briarcliff Junior College with an associate degree on or around 1948. My mother excelled in high school and college as did my father. She was involved in many extracurricular activities and was also a cheerleader. This is interesting because she was the cheerleader for our family and was the glue that kept us together. My mother is in the first row second from right.

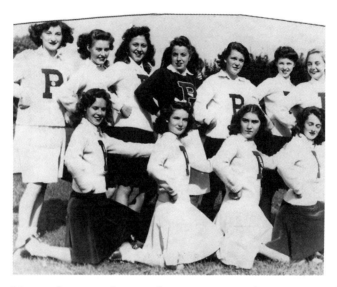

My mother was the comforter, nurturer, listener, complimenter, and mental caregiver my whole life, and she did a great job. I adored her! My father managed the financial aspects of our lives and the cost of caring for Betsy. However, he could not maintain the checkbook, which my mother did; she did a great job balancing the checkbook by hand.

Move to Florida

When my parents retired and moved to Florida in 1987, Betsy came with them, during which time they interacted with her on a daily basis. She moved with them because of the divorce from her first husband, Mark (which I do not have any detail to in-

clude), and because she was experiencing great difficulty dealing
with her illness. However, despite
the fact that my sister ended up
living with them beginning around
1987, my father was not very empathetic or patient, and did not
demonstrate a great deal of compassion when he'd had to interact
with her, but was finally able to
accept the fact that she was truly
mentally ill.

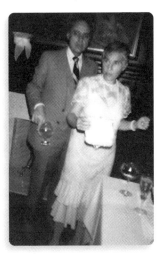

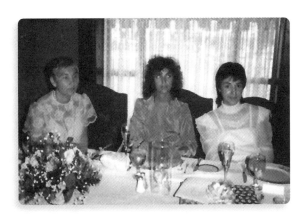

Before the move Betsy had gotten a divorce, after which her
illness worsened. Her wedding to a man named Mark was small
but elegant. As I recall, they were married for fewer than two
years. I do not know much about their relationship because at
the time I was living in Florida and had not seen much of Betsy.

The following picture is the only one I have with my mother and sister together at the reception for Betsy's first marriage, which was in or around 1983.

After Betsy's short-lived first marriage to Mark, my parents did not want to leave her behind when they moved to Ormond Beach, Florida, in 1987, so she went with them. At that time I had already started attending NAMI meetings. I strongly suggested that they attend a chapter in their county, but they never did. However, they read the literature I sent them. They also read a few important and well-written books about the disorder. They were voracious readers, and they learned a great deal. For example, they learned they were not alone, that there were support groups to help families, and that it would be OK when asked to tell close friends about Betsy's illness.

Sadly, but not unexpectedly, the many more years dealing with Betsy's illness finally drained my mother of the emotional stamina to deal with her daughter's highs and lows. At this point, my father and I took over dealing with Betsy, and I continually visited her in the various places she lived and psychiatric hospitals she was admitted to in Florida until she moved to New Jersey in 2001.

As you have read, I highlighted some of the key behaviors of my family. I did this so you will better understand the link between your family background and why past learned and repeated behaviors can have a negative impact on a person afflicted with mental illness and on their family and caretakers. Unfortunately, some people are more reluctant to participate in therapy or unwilling to accept any responsibility to help themselves or their loved one.

My suggestion is to observe the behaviors within your family, get help from professionals, and accept responsibility for your actions toward anyone in your family who is mentally ill. You should also accept that much of your behavior is what you learned from your parents, and you can end the cycle. Once you do this, you will be a step closer to ending the learned and damaging behavior.

Why I Didn't Have Children

I chose not to have children and never looked for a man I could have children with. I never had the burning desire to have children and was more interested in having a career. But the main reason I made this choice was because after years of dealing with my sister's illness and well before I got married in 1990, I had learned more about genetics and the genetic link in my family. A woman I met when I attended NAMI meetings in Boca Raton had been married to a man who was bipolar, and two of her three sons also suffered from the illness. Her family situation was so unusual that she participated in a study at Yale University about family members who have the same illness.

I decided to never bring a child into the world for fear the illness would be passed on to my offspring. The continually strained relationship with my sister also upset me, as I knew that in my golden years I would not have children to become close with but only an abusive sister to care for. I hope that whatever decision any of you make—to have or not have children—you've researched and thought about it.

EVENTS THAT COULD HAVE TRIGGERED THE ILLNESS 02

Overview

When I started to write this book, my thought process focused on memories about my sister, Betsy, and our family background. Betsy experienced several tragic events, which, at the time, I believed were trigger points that brought out her illness. Many of the behaviors she demonstrated when she was a teenager were more prominent after she was diagnosed with bipolar disorder. The events described are first love, drug experimentation, youthful deaths from drug overdoses, frequent moves, attendance at four different universities, and when her life fell apart.

First Love, Drug Experimentation, Friends' Deaths from Drug Overdoses

When my sister was a teenager, she was very energetic and hyper; she moved from activity to activity, changed clothes several times a day, and tidied up her room more than once a day. These behaviors may have been the beginning manifestations of her disorder. My mother's theory was that Betsy's drug use during her teen years was not just for experimentation but to sedate herself from the manic highs. My mother was a very insightful and thoughtful person, and she surmised that because Betsy had no idea what was wrong with her, she used drugs in order to slow down her racing mind. Betsy eventually became a prescription medication abuser, which exacerbated her condition. For example, she was always seeking more medication and painkillers and my mother told me that several pharmacies in Daytona Beach, FL refused to refill her prescriptions

Only when she was in what I would call a sane and logical mood did she admit that she had an addiction problem. Luckily, because she lived in one assisted living facility, Evergreen Court in Spring Valley, New York, from 2008 to when it burned to the ground in 2021, her medications were tightly controlled. However, she was always seeking medication (e.g., painkillers). One of her strategies was to tell the staff that her back hurt and she needed to go the hospital, and there she would receive the pain medication.

It was during her first year in high school, when she was about fourteen years old (at that time we lived in a suburb of Pittsburgh, Pennsylvania, in Upper Saint Clair Township), that I remember her starting to experiment with drugs. She had a boyfriend, Bob (deceased), whom my parents disapproved of.

When they were dating, they both experimented with marijuana, hashish, and (I believe) heroin and alcohol. She often smoked pot in her bedroom or came home stoned.

While my sister was living at home after she graduated from high school in 1972 and was attending the University of Massachusetts, Dartmouth (in the 1970s it was called Southeastern Massachusetts University), she dated another man who was involved in drugs. This might have been another trigger point that enhanced her illness, which prior to 1975 was undiagnosed. He, like many other men she dated, was from a very wealthy family and could afford the drugs. She immersed herself in this unhealthy relationship; she would come home stoned and would tell me what they had done. My father would not allow him in the house, even though my father knew his parents; they were members of the same country club. The man was named Rocky. His father was a prominent gynecologist, and his mother was a wealthy heiress. He and his brother were wild teenagers, drove fast cars, drank, and partied a great deal. As I recall, Rocky was the oldest and had dropped out of college. Betsy resented my dad for not allowing Rocky in the house.

I learned later that in the 1970s doing drugs was considered to be part of the maturation process many teens experienced. Drugs are also one of the fads teens get involved in, but for my sister, I don't believe experimenting with drugs was ever a fad. It was her escape from the realities of her life. For these men the purpose was probably for the high, but for my sister drugs served two purposes: to get high and to sedate her uncontrollable and bizarre thought patterns and moods.

Youthful Deaths Due to Drug Overdoses

Betsy's first love was with a teenager, Bob, who lived in Upper Saint Clair Township, which is south of Pittsburgh, Pennsylvania. They were crazy about each other. My father did not allow her to finish her senior year in high school and required her to move to Massachusetts.

Her relationship with Bob caused what I recall was the first major riff between my father and her, which continued through the rest of her life. My father did not want her dating him and didn't allow him in the house. So for their entire relationship, before we moved to Massachusetts, she saw him secretly. She voiced her hatred for our father for forcing her to move away and leave Bob. She was also quite upset about leaving her very close high school friends in her senior year. But most of all, she had lost her first love. I know many women do not marry their first love, but for my sister, he was the ultimate.

For several years after we had moved, she kept Bob's pictures in her jewelry box or wallet. Additionally, one of her best friends ended up dating him. This was also very upsetting to her despite the fact that she no longer lived in Pennsylvania. But what an irony that despite being from an affluent family and able to do anything with his life, several years after we moved away, he died of a drug overdose. Betsy was devastated. The fact that he was her first love may have worsened her later condition, because she, like many people, did not handle death well. Several years later her best girlfriend, Loraine, from the same town (with whom she stayed in touch), had moved to Hollywood, Florida. She, too, died of a drug overdose. I know that Betsy's loss of close friends and both deaths had an adverse effect on her. I know she was extremely sad, cried a great deal, and was despondent.

Frequent Moves and Attendance at Four Universities

My father began working for Goodyear Rubber and Tire Corporation in 1950 and worked his way up the hierarchy. As I mentioned earlier, we moved a great deal. He spent much of his time traveling for business, and when he was home, he was on the golf course, with my mother, or with his friends, but not with us. When he was around, it was my sister who managed to get what little attention he was able to give. I was just a nuisance and a loudmouth. My mother also worked, and she tried to be the mediator, but she (I strongly feel) also favored my sister, although less than my father did. I had a slight weight problem, was very flat chested, and was considered the weaker and less intelligent child who lacked focus, and my slim sister was considered the brain, the achiever, the better test taker, and the one with a better figure and physical agility. My parents never directly stated this to my face, but there were subtle implications. Moreover, my sister made fun of me because of my flat chest and was critical of my swimming and weak physical agility.

When my father accepted another promotional opportunity in the state of Massachusetts, as noted previously, Betsy was forced to leave her peer group during her senior year of high school.

This accelerated her dislike of my father. She eventually adapted very well to the new environment. She made many friends who were on the same intellectual level she was, and the friendships were, in part, based on their mutual behavior of smoking pot.

She dove heavily into her books as an escape, and initially she didn't have a solid peer group. The people were generally very cliquey at our new high school, and even though we made new friends, Betsy no longer held the same status she had at her prior high school.

As most of you will probably recall, the peer group one establishes in high school is especially important to teenagers. Being uprooted from a particularly important peer group, which many times has more influence on a person than their family, is not easy. It wasn't for my sister. Each time we moved, we both resented my father for uprooting us. My sister's resentment of my father was significantly greater than mine.

I also believe that another way she handled all the changes she was experiencing, including becoming manic or depressed, was using mild drugs in high school and college. Whenever she was home, she would listen to the stereo and would quite frequently smoke pot. She also smoked pot whenever my parents were not at home. Her resentment toward my parents was evident even during her teens, and unfortunately it continued to deteriorate as the years went on. She'd constantly criticize them, no matter what they did to try to help her. It didn't matter if she was stoned or not. Nothing was ever good enough.

I believe that because Betsy had a boyfriend (Bob) she adored whom she was torn away from, she started to use more drugs to fight off what was going on in her mind and because she missed him so much. We moved from Pennsylvania in 1972, and she had her drug overdose in 1975.

Although Betsy wasn't officially diagnosed with bipolar

disorder until age nineteen, the events that occurred before her diagnosis were more difficult to deal with and grew progressively worse. Examples were bizarre social behavior, attendance at four different universities (she was never happy at the current one), and sexual encounters with many boyfriends. I strongly believe that one of the reasons she attended many different universities was because she was running away from, and in denial about, being diagnosed with bipolar disorder.

After already attending two schools (one was Arizona State University) and checking out a third (during the years 1973 to 1977), she decided to head to Florida State University. While she was with my cousin Kim in Arizona, they went out to the desert and were joy riding in a dune buggy. Kim's fiancé was killed instantly in a crash. I do not know details of the crash other than it was a horrible scene. As my parents and I recalled, Betsy was very troubled by this and returned home. During the approximately two years she spent with my now-deceased first cousin Kim in Arizona and on World Campus Afloat, they became very close. But she lost another person close to her after the death of Kim's fiancé. Shortly thereafter, Kim went to Mexico for several months, met members of the Unification Church at an airport or somewhere in Phoenix, and joined the cult. Betsy never saw or heard from her again and was sad.

By this time in Betsy's life, one of her best friends, Loraine; a boyfriend, Bob (the same Bob discussed earlier); and then her first cousin, Kim, died. While Betsy was living in Spring Valley, New York, Kim was living in Rhinebeck, New York, with her family. Betsy made several attempts to see Kim, but Kim never responded. Her brother, Michael, told me that she did not want to see Betsy because she was afraid that Betsy would ask her for money, which she could not spare. Betsy was upset that Kim did not want to reconnect with her after so many years. When I told Betsy that Kim had died from breast cancer, she did not seem to be too concerned. However, overall, Betsy did not handle death well, and I always thought about this. I wondered if the deaths exacerbated her illness.

Betsy's college years were full of mental turmoil. Can you imagine yourself going to four universities in five years in four different states, and summer school in two different states? Each time you would have to start over. I recall that she didn't like any of the universities she was attending at that moment and did what she could to go elsewhere. Bipolar individuals operate from the moment, from whatever fits their needs and feelings at the time. Betsy demonstrated that behavior her entire life and was fortunate that my parents were financially able to pay for all her changes. Thinking back over the years, I realized that she was trying to escape her mania and weird thoughts and hoped that a different environment and school would make her well.

As I said earlier, Betsy's illness manifested itself in 1975. She had been in several unhealthy relationships with men, including Rocky, whom she did drugs with in high school. My father was afraid for her safety, particularly because she stayed out very late with him many nights, and he drove a fancy, fast Audi convertible. When she came home, she was usually very stoned and out of it. He was several years her senior, had already graduated from college, and was not doing anything with his life.

I surmise that he was being supported by his parents. Overall, he was not a good influence on her. Once she graduated from high school and went to college, she never saw him again. My father was very happy about this.

One of Betsy's letters, on the next page, partially describes her struggle with new medications and the effects they were having on her teeth. Despite all the sadness in her letter, she did write down some goals. She also expressed her fear of losing my mother, at which point, over the phone, I assured her I would always be there for her.

Dear Linsey,

How are you and Frank & the cats? I really wish I could see you all - we should arrange a way for me to visit.

I don't know if I told you but I am back on Desryl. Now I can sleep 8 hrs. and it's already helping as an antidepressant. I have to have tons of work on my teeth - they look awful and hurt but in a few months they'll be all done and looking good. Back in a minute. I'm re reading an excellent physiological psychology book - unbelievable!

My AC is getting fixed this afternoon - Thank god. I'm getting my food stamps application under-way finally - I had to get a new

Social Security card.

You know what I need is a car soon so mummy doesn't have to run here all the time. What will I do if something happens to her ?! Daddy doesn't understand the first thing about my situation. Please come visit me or let me come visit you so we can talk.

I'm listening to geraldo, I'm gonna walk read, eat later. I eat very healthy food and do 15 mi. on the bike once or twice daily with a hand weight.

2 nice looking guys w/ money asked me out but dumped me. I am hurt but relieved. I care the most about sleep, no AIDS, health, getting better, friends and improving my mind and the apartment and somehow getting a part time job for a phone and car. Love you ! Betsy

Families of people with mental illness face many stresses—financial burdens, emotional upheaval, and practical problems of living with someone who is seriously ill. Families are not the cause of mental illness. Most can benefit from the support of other family members through self-help groups such as the National Alliance for the Mentally Ill.[10]

When Betsy's Life Fell Apart

After her first marriage to Mark ended, Betsy had extraordinarily little security in her life. For example, she never established any permanent roots. She moved from Massachusetts to Connecticut, Connecticut to Arizona, Arizona to Massachusetts, Massachusetts to Florida, Florida to Pennsylvania, Pennsylvania to Florida, Florida to New Jersey, and then finally settled in New York for the last eighteen or so years of her life. After she left the secure world of academia and received a master of social work degree (with a concentration on psychiatric social work) from the University of Pennsylvania, she had a boyfriend, full-time jobs, and some stability.

After the stability in Betsy's life ended, and around the time of her first short-lived marriage and subsequent divorce, her illness worsened. At that time, I recall she was no longer taking lithium and a mild tranquilizer. Her mood cycles were more frequent, and the highs and lows were more pronounced. My parents and I learned much later that she was diagnosed as a rapid cycler. This type of disorder entails twenty-four hours of mania or depression and twenty-four hours of the opposite and

---

10. NAMI brochure, 1993.

is very difficult to stabilize. Unfortunately, after her first marriage and divorce, her only option was to move back home with my parents, and during this time Betsy would sleepwalk. My mother told me that she would find Betsy walking and totally asleep. My mom would also hear shuffling or walking noises outside her bedroom, would jump out of bed, and would find Betsy walking and be totally asleep. This occurred more than once, and one time my mother got there just in time to keep Betsy from falling down the stairs. The year was 1986 before my parents moved to Florida. They found another psychiatrist for her to see, and I am quite sure she was prescribed new medications.

Fortunately, she had been stable for almost nine years because she was taking lithium and a tranquilizer, she had stability in her life, a boyfriend, constant intellectual stimulation in graduate school, a full-time position in her field, no financial worries, and a wonderful place to live. Her stability for approximately nine years does not erase the fact that the years after her first marriage and divorce were horrific for her and for me and my parents. From that point on, we picked up the pieces of her shattered life, and we walked on eggshells.

As noted previously, my sister moved home with my parents after the divorce from her first husband in or around 1985. After moving to Florida in 1987, she had greater difficulty dealing with the manic highs and dark and gloomy lows, and had to change the jobs she held in social work a number of times because she was fighting the illness. I continually scouted the Sunday papers for her and continued to send her newspaper clippings. She applied for a PhD program in Florida (although I forget which university), and although she was rejected, I think that this was her last-ditch attempt to do something with her life, something that would help her escape the terror of the illness that was stealing her life away. Betsy even lived with me in Florida for a few months in 1988, but it was exhausting and didn't work out. She ran around after the men in my condominium complex, stayed out late, and was verbally abusive to me whenever she was in a black mood. She moved back in with my parents, who lived in Ormond Beach, Florida.

Eventually, my mother helped her apply for Social Security Disability benefits in 1989, and Betsy resigned herself to a life without work. She was very sad about this because she would not be using her education, nor would she have a successful and interesting career. However, she frequently talked and wrote about the day that she would work again in her field.

No matter what Betsy did, she failed and ended up back where she started: no work, no man, and having lost all the new friends she made. Over many years, from 1989 to 2001, she shoplifted, had Baker Act hearings (a Baker Act is when a person is involuntarily committed to a psychiatric hospital or medical unit of a jail), had marriages and divorces, told pathological lies, hit a police officer, threatened to kill my father, wrecked a car, experienced numerous other minor fender benders, had repeated evictions from apartment complexes, continually abused medication, physically attacked my mother, hit a blind man, drank while on medication, had stays in jail, completed a three-month dual-diagnosis program, stole medication from an adult congregate living facility (ACLF), tested positive for illegal drug use in an ACLF, and tested positive for cocaine—all of which can be partially explained by the many sad and horrific characteristics of a person who has bipolar disorder. Life became a failure for her.

I cannot recall the number of times I would cry about Betsy's life when I was alone or when my mother and I were sitting together. We wished her life would get better.

If you have a bipolar relative, child, parent, or spouse, some of these incidents might sound familiar. But even if your experience has not been as terrible as the aforementioned, becoming familiar with the characteristics will provide you with a better understanding of the personality disorder. Be prepared to expect the unexpected. These behaviors might seem unbelievable to those not afflicted with this disorder. It is so difficult for the unafflicted to understand what mentally ill people go through, and each case is unique and different. Please read the above paragraph again and try to understand their plight. My sister was not the worst, nor was she the best case. Again, please be prepared, as best you can, for the unexpected. The next section summarizes and provides examples of many of my sister's characteristics.

THE CHARACTERISTICS 03

Overview

The first section in this chapter summarizes some information about the disorder from the DSM-5, which is the diagnostic and statistical manual psychiatrists and psychotherapists use to diagnose mental disorders. It is used by health care professionals throughout the United States and standardizes the language they use to communicate with and about their patients.[11]

Numerous characteristics are described in this chapter and were not obtained from an academic textbook on the disorder. Each of the characteristics I write about came from my mind, what I recalled and experienced when with my sister, over the phone, or through letters. In addition, I have some personal experience with people I have known who were also afflicted with bipolar disorder or depression. The list of characteristics is too long to include here; nonetheless, each one is described below in vivid detail. Betsy's letters and cards are included to

---

11. Jessica Trushcel, "Bipolar Definition and DSM-5 Diagnostic Criteria," Remedy Health Media, LLC, https://www.psycom.net/bipolar-definition-dsm-5.

validate my descriptions, and suggestions for how you can deal with similar situations are included in most sections.

Academic Descriptions of Different Types of Bipolar Disorder

As I learned over the years, but was unable to describe in an intelligent manner, there are different forms of bipolar disorder. The three very different forms are:

- Bipolar I Disorder, which is characterized with or without psychotic episodes
- Bipolar II Disorder, which is less severe depression or mania, does not prevent someone from functioning, and can alternate between both states
- Cyclothymic Disorder, which is cyclical in nature, in which the episodes of depression and mania are brief[12]

The academic definition is "a group of brain disorders that cause extreme fluctuation in a person's mood, energy, and ability to function," which describes my sister perfectly. However, the academic descriptions from the DSM-5 of the various symptoms of depression and mania also describe my sister's behavior. Without having read any definitions from the DSM-5 until I was finishing this book, the characteristics described in this chapter are much the same. The list of hypomanic characteristics from the DSM-5 are:

---

12. Jessica Trushcel, "Bipolar Definition."

- inflated self-esteem or grandiosity
- decreased need for sleep
- increased talkativeness
- racing thoughts
- distracted easily
- increased goal-directed activity or psychomotor agitation
- engaging in activities that hold the potential for painful consequences (e.g., unrestrained buying sprees)[13]

It is interesting to note that four of these characteristics—decreased need for sleep; increased talkativeness; being distracted easily; and increase in goal-directed activity or psychomotor agitation—are behaviors that my sister demonstrated frequently but that did not have an adverse effect on me in terms of the pain and sorrow she caused when she demonstrated the other characteristics.

However, I did mention that Betsy would sleepwalk, and I know that she had difficulty getting to sleep at night. Also, when she was in a manic state, she did talk fast and, at times, rushed around and cleaned up anything that was out of order or not to her liking. Many times, when I went to visit Betsy at Evergreen Court, Spring Valley, New York, she would be so excited to see me that she would immediately ask me to take her shopping and would pressure me a great deal until I called a cab and took her shopping. After shopping she would want

---

13. Jessica Trushcel, "Bipolar Definition."

to go out to eat and then stop at another store or place on the way back to Evergreen Court.

Also, regarding a decreased need for sleep, this often happened when I was visiting with Betsy. We would spend several hours together, and then she would be very tired and take a nap. An example of how she was easily distracted is that she would run up and down the halls, in and outside the lobby at Evergreen Court, and then finally sit down when she went to smoke a cigarette. Sometimes I could not keep up with her and would just sit down somewhere and chat with one or more of the residents.

The DSM-5 list of depressed states of mind are as follows:

- depressed mood most of the day, nearly every day
- loss of interest or pleasure in all, or almost all, activities
- significant weight loss or decrease or increase in appetite
- engaging in purposeless movements, such as pacing the room
- fatigue or loss of energy
- feelings of worthlessness or guilt
- diminished ability to think or concentrate, or indecisiveness
- recurrent thoughts of death, recurrent suicidal ideation without a specific plan, or a suicide attempt.[14]

---

14. Jessica Trushcel, "Bipolar Definition."

Of these, engaging in purposeless movements or pacing, fatigue or loss of energy, and diminished ability to think are not included as one of the characteristics described in this chapter. I did observe each one in Betsy's behavior, but none caused me great pain or sorrow.

In summary, I want anyone who is a medical or health professional and is reading the next section of this book to understand that I did not write as nor am I presenting myself as an expert in the field, but rather as a layperson who has had a great deal of experience dealing with my sister's illness.

Periods of Mania and Depression

With all our personal problems, it is difficult to walk in the shoes of a person suffering from bipolar disorder. Throughout Betsy's life she was either very manic or extremely depressed. A few of her letters best describe what she was experiencing, and if you are suffering from a similar illness, please reflect on your life.

Dear Limse,

I am really hypomanic sick and my phone isn't working — battery only partially charging. I cleaned everything and found 2 more suitcases that Drew sent me (set of 7 altogether) navy. Boy it makes me want to visit you but absolutely no money and now no sanity. I'll be able to put a partial payment on the phone bill. Joe was very abusive yesterday which didn't help my condition. Reading, writing + cleaning helps. I am almost full blown manic so it really is better if I'm not cooped up. My disc player + phone are fucked up and I bet Joe did it altho' he's not known to do that before. He usually gives things. Well all this has lead to no coffee, no cigs.

I really should pull away from Joe completely + now's the time to do it when the phone's fucked up. I love my phone – it keeps me company and the caller ID and call waiting is cool, too. My friend Bob just bought a turbo car so I can ask him for rides plus he gets food stamps so in a day or so maybe everything will get fixed. I'm walking over to Cobblestone after I get fixed up (hair!) people moving out gave me some nice healthy plants. I don't want to leave my room – I feel I'm coming down a little. Now Joe won't be able to contact me. Ha. Ha. I wish I could go to the tanning salon. I call the bank everyday for exact balance. I'm pretty dizzy on and off. Boy did I do a good cleaning job and I'm gonna donate some stuff in a bag, too.

Dear Linsey + Frank,

I am very sad and in pain because after the manic episode is the dull depression. BuT! I can foresee bringing more good things into my life this time and having more say so about good things happening to me. We are the masters of our own fate. I do feel ready to work part time and even I wonder if I'll ever get good help anymore; but, the nurses say I'm doing better and better each day, Drew calls often - he's really hung up on going back to night school but his aspirations are always unrealistic. Right now he has a decent job + no expenses. Boy, I wish I had a card or a plant or flowers from you. Mom brought pj's, books + good cheer. I still love my apartment and the strange social life of the pool. I love the tanning salon too. I'm dying to buy some shoes, 2 outfits wax my eyebrows, maybe get a kitty & start working out (2 hrs day!) For the 8th time I had PMS then came to the hospital & got my period. I need a *goof* endocrinologist. I'm sleepy & feel full from spaghetti. I better not gain an ounce — I'm 120 now,

Love Belsy
Write / Call!

Betsy was a rapid cycler with bipolar disorder, which is the most difficult to stabilize. Although the term rapid cycler does not appear on the previous list, both she and my mother told me that this is what she was told by different medical professionals. As I saw it, her life was like riding on a roller coaster every day, one which would go fast, slow down, go fast again, and go uphill and rapidly downhill. During the rides she was manic or depressed and would demonstrate very bizarre behavior and actions that would hurt her and alienate the people who were the recipients. Even with their knowledge and experience, on more than one occasion, my parents used the Baker Act to force her to be hospitalized and locked down. In so doing, I believe they saved her life.

Verbal Abuse

I have many flashbacks about growing up with Betsy, with whom I believe I never had a normal, ongoing, healthy relationship. My remembrances of my sister's verbal abuse are that it often put me in a deeply sad mood, even though it was just temporary. To her, I was a "loudmouthed, smelly, fat, and ugly lesbian." I recall there were very few times, while growing up with my sister, when she was nice to me. Her verbal abuse was part of the illness; I believe that she viewed me as what she was expected to become. If your loved one verbally abuses you, try to throw the pain over your shoulder and out of your mind, even if it requires tremendous energy.

A very memorable incident occurred during the late 1960s, when we were living in Huntington, Long Island, New York.

Some of Betsy's actions and behavior may have been the beginning of her bipolar disorder. Both of us were in elementary school. I was sharing a double bed with my sister because whenever my maternal grandmother, Reva, was visiting from Arizona, we shared a room. I received a kick in my legs, was told I stank, and was pushed out of bed onto the floor. I remember getting up and moving to the couch in the living room. The physical and emotional pain enveloped me, and I was unable to move for a few hours. I did not understand why she was so verbally abusive and kicked me out of the bed.

As mentioned previously, Betsy was very athletic. She auditioned for the gymnastics team and made it, but I did not. She was a borderline genius, and popular with both men and women. I always had difficulty reconciling that her disorder destroyed her life. The best way to describe it was that I lived in her shadow. It was difficult to not compare myself to Betsy: she made all As, and I didn't; she aced algebra, trigonometry, and calculus, and I didn't; she was the faster swimmer, could do gymnastics, always had a boyfriend, and I didn't.

Growing up and throughout my life, I was in her shadow both before and after her illness. When I compared myself to Betsy (which of course, I should have not done), at times that comparison made me very sad. Because her verbal abuse contributed to my low self-esteem, I always thought that I was not as smart, attractive, athletic, or creative (and other adjectives I need not list) as she. My mother used to tell me, "Linsey, you are a late bloomer and will find success much later in life." And although she was correct, the repetitive comment did not help my self-esteem.

I opine that our life experiences stay with us throughout our lifetime. They impact us positively or negatively as to how we deal with life. Examples from my lived experiences include not repeating the same mistakes, changing my perceptions when I needed to, constantly learning, and adding value to my work, my husband and friends, and particularly my sister's life. When anyone has a close family member who is suffering from a crippling mental illness, their life experience will be far different than if the person were not an integral part of their life. Unbelievably, the mentally ill person can enrich a person's life. In my case, the poor treatment I received from my sister helped make me a better person and an excellent caregiver to her. I tried to forgive her for all the years of verbal abuse.

A summary of some of her verbal and general abuse includes the following:

- name calling
- totally ignoring me
- making fun of the size of my breasts
- telling me I stunk
- taking advantage of my kindness and generosity
- verbally lashing out whenever I tried to correct or stop her behavior
- hitting and scratching
- picking a fight
- constant belittling

My first therapist taught me to not focus on the old *if, and, but, and should have been* syndrome. Unfortunately, I could not change what was. But over many agonizing and painful years thinking about and speaking with Betsy on the phone and seeing her in person, I learned to remind myself that I did not cause the behavior and could not change what had happened.

Today, I know that part of what motivated me was attributable to Betsy's verbal abuse. Much pain and sorrow, I believe, drove me to go on, never quit, and accomplish a great deal.

One redeeming quality (which is undoubtedly one of the reasons I never abandoned Betsy) was that she created and sent me many beautiful cards and letters over the years, which, in a way, compensated for the past damage to my ego and self-esteem. No matter what she did, how she behaved, or how grueling it was to deal with a traumatic experience in person, I was always there for her. Betsy was my sister, and I loved her, despite how poorly she treated me.

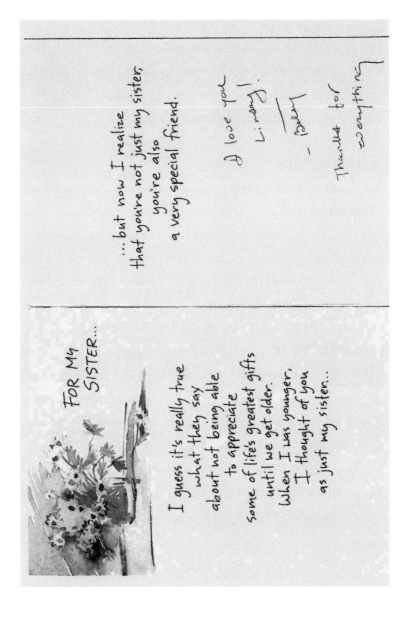

FOR MY
SISTER...

I guess it's really true
what they say
about not being able
to appreciate
some of life's greatest gifts
until we get older.
When I was younger,
I thought of you
as just my sister...

...but now I realize
that you're not just my sister,
you're also
a very special friend.

I love you,
Lindsay!

— Brenda

Thanks for
everything.

Throughout my life with Betsy, I continued to ask myself, "Is this her true personality, or is her awful and abusive behavior one characteristic of the illness and partially caused by the medications?" Overall, despite how badly she treated me with her constant verbal abuse, I survived and continued to build my self-esteem and was always there for her.

A Racing Mind

Betsy had difficulty analyzing, synthesizing, and processing information in a logical sequence and slowing down her mind, and constantly changed subjects when talking to me. Because she was thinking so many thoughts at once, and at such a fast pace, her mind would become fogged up, and then, sometimes, she would crash into a depressed state. My sister explained it this way: "My thoughts race, and it feels as if my head is going to explode." Her racing mind was reflected in many of her long letters, in which she wrote on many topics in one paragraph.

Her mind raced when she was in a manic phase, and then she would abuse her medications and become ill. She also periodically had terrible migraine headaches.

The letter on the next page provides an example of how her mind raced, changing subjects a great deal and making commentary about her living situation and not getting high.

Dear Lindsey,

Look! I got some pretty stationary. I colored my hair but maybe too much. Mom's due over today for the doctor's appts and a two evenings. Thank God she does my bedies/laundry too or it comes out w/ bleach or not at all. I made 4 necklaces and have 8 ornative and Dan't to do 3 or 4 xmas team - miniatures. Don't forget my lists. on the calendar it says you've cared more busy than any friend ever could, yes, Lindsey Thank you for your compassion,

I dislike everyone here except some of the staff. You walk on the bears + feel it's so grimy. I feel so up and down about what I can gain from here. I like the money goodies and special treatment I get because they trust me and my clean, I haven't gotten high since Jan. so I get a pardon soon and $10.00 shopping. I finally bought a watch but I don't know if it's water proof when I swim. I haven't gotten high and mean no joke, I didn't drink anyday but I will try the water a few times. It's water under the bridge. Again I want writing, reading + ways to keep to work on in my room because if I stay in my room I don't get

Making irrational decisions often occurred during a manic phase. For example, Betsy had difficulty delaying gratification, and as a result, when we went shopping, she would load the shopping cart up with items I knew she did not need, and when I would gently tell her that she needed to be more selective, she would yell or scream at me. During a manic phase, Betsy was not cognizant of the consequences of her actions and lived only for the moment. My parents and I were always picking up the pieces of whatever problem she caused.

At times Betsy would break out in a terrible skin rash, which I believe was stress related, and one time she suffered from shingles. Whenever this happened, I wondered if the stress of her racing mind triggered the physical medical conditions.

If your child or friend is experimenting with drugs, has a tendency to be constantly active, and exhibits bizarre, uncontrollable, and agitated behavior, they might be experiencing a manic episode. Also, if they have trouble sleeping, this is a sign that they may be depressed or too manic to sleep. During a manic phase, they may talk quickly and incessantly about their plans, ideas, people, or how they feel. When Betsy's mind was racing, she would become scared because she could not control her actions and did not remember what took place.

One of the most upsetting and debilitating situations was when she was involved with a man who also suffered from a mental disorder. She met one in the psychiatric ward of a hospital in Saint Augustine, Florida, sometime between 1990 and 1993. They moved in together. He was a recovered alcoholic, was on disability, and told her that he became an alcoholic to sedate himself. He had not been diagnosed with a mental disorder, and because of his alcoholism, he could not finish his premed college degree. Sadly, the disease took control of his hopes for a normal, prosperous life. I do not recall his name.

I was hopeful that their relationship would last, because they had similar life experiences and could help each other. How wrong I was.

He was a genuinely nice man who was struggling hard to make a life for himself with some part-time work and his disability check. When receiving disability payments, you are only allowed to work a certain number of hours and make only a limited amount of money before the benefits are curtailed. The system works against people with mental disorders because the disability checks are just barely enough to live on (i.e., the annual stipend doesn't bring a person above the poverty line), and in many states the resources are scarce.

Betsy checked herself out of the hospital against all medical advice, which was poor judgment. She became very aggressive and was marked by an impulse to commit suicide. Based on my recollection, she physically attacked him. He could not control her and called the police. When they arrived, she went after one officer and was subsequently arrested and charged with assaulting a police officer.

The bail was over $5,000, and my parents would not pay it. It was their decision. At the time I thought that the mentally ill did not belong in a regular county jail. Despite the fact that the authorities knew of her mental disorder they would not put her in a hospital. Instead, they locked her in a jail cell for close to six months with little or no exercise. I do not recall whether they gave her medication. I was not present during this horrific and sad time, but my parents told me that no one seemed to care that my sister was mentally ill.

My first emotion was anger because my father chose not to pay the $5,000 bail. But he hoped—and my mother and I agreed—that the time in jail would give Betsy time to reflect. It was an environment where her medications would be strictly controlled, and she might learn from the incident. Many years later, whenever I thought about that situation, I realized how ignorant we were about her illness, because we were critical that she did not learn from her mistakes. She could not learn from her mistakes, because while she was involved in the situation, she had no control over her actions and then did not recall what transpired.

During her incarceration, my parents, once again, had to pick up the broken pieces of her life, in this case, removing her belongings and apologizing to the man and his parents. Once my sister was released from jail, my mother had to find her somewhere else to live. My sister blamed others and wouldn't admit she was drinking heavily or that the drugs mixed with the alcohol caused the problem.

After Betsy was released from jail, the police would not send her to a psychiatric hospital. During this period in her life, she still had resiliency and stamina—enough that she was able to move forward. In hindsight it might have been positive that she did not recall the events that caused her to lose her boyfriend and go to jail.

When she was released from jail, she just moved on to another phase of her illness and to a new place to live. However, she never spent another day in jail, but I cannot attribute this to any learning that took place. How can learning take place when the person does not recollect what transpired before, during, and after an incident over which they have no control? It may have just been repressed.

Bizarre Social Behavior

Another indispensable point is that if you are a parent or sibling, be cautious of overly bizarre behavior. This might be an important sign that something is not quite right. During Betsy's teen years, we knew there was something not quite right, but we attributed it to drug usage, which was the cool thing to do in the 1970s, hanging out with spoiled, rich boys and girls who had no direction and had things handed to them on a silver platter.

As noted previously, my sister demonstrated a great deal of bizarre social behavior during manic or depressed states. Some specific examples include the following:

- giving away her possessions to newly acquired friends
- stealing money from others' purses
- constantly changing her clothes
- chugging beverages
- asking you for one of your belongings that she wanted

- ordering more food for one meal than one person could possibly eat and not finishing the food—we were at an Italian restaurant in Nanuet, New York, and Betsy had to order two entrees

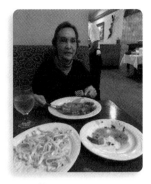

- interrupting others when they are talking
- flirting with someone else's spouse
- walking up to a complete stranger and making positive or negative comments to them
- grabbing something out of your hands

When Betsy appeared to be stable, not manic or depressed, she was fun to be around and could carry on a normal and, many times, very intellectual conversation. But our discussions evolved to ones that were mainly about her and her out-of-place priorities, such as going to the tanning salon, going shopping for clothes that she did not need, etcetera.

Her relationships with both woman friends and men she was dating often ended abruptly. Anytime a new friendship ended, she implied that it was because the person or persons were low class, losers, were uneducated, drug users, etcetera. She had negative encounters with people, sometimes labeling a woman "malicious," though a normal person would not conclude that about them. Betsy could not deal with stress in any relationship. Stress was triggered when I questioned her. On the other hand, so many of the nurses, CNAs, doctors, and other health professionals I spoke to over the phone or met in person commented on how nice, smart, funny, and interesting Betsy was. None of them ever complained to me about her.

You should research the medication prescribed to your family member. You should also ascertain which behaviors are manifestations of over- or underuse of medication.

Bizarre social behavior is a trait of people with bipolar disorder. Based on what I have observed, side effects, contra-indications, and misuse of medication caused some of Betsy's bizarre behavior. Under- or overuse of medications can also cause nasty side effects; for example, the person may become more irritable and moodier than their normal state and take it out on their loved ones or friends.

My sister told me many times that she never knew when she would go off into one of her uncontrollable manic episodes, and that was the reason she checked herself into the hospital. She desperately wanted to be in control of her actions and mind. I cannot provide an exact count of the number of times she did this, but I suspect it was well over seventy-five times. To her, a manic episode was like being high on cocaine. She had used the drug in the past, and when she did, she thought she was invincible, was extremely confident, was hyperalert, and could say anything she wanted to anyone, regardless of the circumstance.

In summary, as tragic, shocking, stressful, and outrageous as her behavior was, I learned to live with it. However, over the years, there were times when the incidents I was willing and able to effectively deal with took a toll on me. For example, I would often mentally beat myself up, because I thought I had done something wrong. After so many years of Betsy blaming me for anything bad that happened to her, I became conditioned. During and after being part of or observing Betsy's bizarre behavior, I always reminded myself that her life would have been much worse if I wasn't there for her during the highs and lows. This is often what family members do to help a child, parent, or sibling who is ill.

Pathological Lying

Based on my research of aberrant personalities, both criminal and noncriminal, I learned that pathological lying is a characteristic of many mental disorders. Considering this, Betsy could not control her lying, but this did not make it any easier for the listener. One lie would be told, and another one would follow to cover up the previous lie.

One lie she told repeatedly was that she was not over- or undermedicating. At the residence where she lived the longest, Evergreen Court in Spring Valley, New York, I do not believe a month would go by when she would not call to tell me that someone had stolen some of her belongings. Smoking in the rooms was forbidden, yet on more than one occasion, she was caught smoking. She would vehemently deny smoking and then accuse the administration of lying to her sister. When an administrator spoke to me, I would plead with them to not make her move or put her out on the street. The only reason they did not evict her was because the state of New York does not allow people like my sister to be evicted without a place to live.

Having learned that pathological liars continue the behavior, I tolerated it for years. She lied to protect her ego and self-esteem, was subconsciously cognizant of the problems she caused herself and others, and would lie, which included blaming others and denying that she had done anything wrong.

Betsy lied often about being a drug abuser or medication seeking, and I believe she did this to cover up her mistakes and to protect her damaged ego.

To save herself from what transpired as a result of her actions, Betsy would create different versions of the same incident. Since she had no control over this behavior, she could and would lie.

People who have an internal locus of control can look at themselves in the mirror and be self-reflective about their problems or issues and attempt to solve them. Those with an external locus of control blame others and environmental factors for their problems or issues. Because of Betsy's illness, she was unable to solve her problems, many of which she created. In her mind, I believe that Betsy had difficulty looking at herself in the mirror because of how the illness ruined the life she could have lived.

Poor Judgment and Decision Making

Poor judgment is a tragic characteristic because of the havoc that ensues, causing adverse effects on many people. Betsy had a pattern of calling for an ambulance when something went wrong. She may have been escaping to the hospital to hide away from the world. Betsy's poor judgment included spending what little money she had on perfume, costume jewelry, or other people; losing money; making emergency phone calls when there wasn't an emergency; and shoplifting and stealing things from other residents' rooms or trying to do so.

Many of the decisions Betsy made were flawed. I believe this was because her mental processing was disordered and tangled and sticky, like a spider's web, affecting her judgment and decision making.

One time in the 1990s, when she was still able to work, she became romantically involved with her boss at the psychiatric hospital where she was employed as a social worker. She immersed herself in her work and loved it, but her inappropriate relationship with her boss resulted in her leaving the position. I do not know if she was fired or left voluntarily.

One time, Betsy was ordered by the court to check herself into a dual-diagnosis treatment center located in Moultrie, Georgia. She decided to check herself out of the facility against medical advice and then spent $250 on a cab ride back to Palatka, Florida, where she was living at the time. I received a call from a bank agent, who said he needed my permission to release $250 from my parents' account, on which I had signature authority. I initially said no but was then told that she needed to pay the cab driver waiting outside the bank. I had no choice but to release the money, because she could have been arrested for nonpayment.

Many times over the years, when I had recovered from one of Betsy's bad judgements or decision-making mishaps, I would recall a horrible experience I had with a friend who was bipolar.

I may have thought about her to fool myself into thinking that Betsy's situation was much better. In fact, over the years, it became worse than the story I am about to tell.

When I was living in Miami, Florida, from 1980 to 1984, this friend was bipolar and told me she had been stable for over twelve years. She was employed as a paralegal and graduated from the University of Pennsylvania. She told me she wanted to do more with her life but could not because of her illness. She told me she was stable because doctors found the "miracle drug combination" for her: Tegretol and lithium.

We went on a vacation to one of the Club Med properties in the Caribbean. It turned out that my friend was manic the whole time. She stayed up all night and locked me out of the room one night while she was in the room having sex with a man she had chased while running nude on the beach. Later, she accused me of stealing the belongings she had apparently left behind at Club Med and was very verbally abusive.

During that unforgettable vacation, I thought, "I'm so glad my sister's illness isn't this bad." Little did I know that I had spoken too soon. My friend had been on a roller coaster for about twelve years, prior to our vacation, before she finally was stabilized. Betsy, my sister, was stable for nine years, and then her entire life fell to pieces. You will never know when it is going to occur for your loved one. It could be any time.

I have always asked myself this question: "Are the poor judgment and decision making side effects of the drug mixtures, combined with the person's lack of self-control and feelings of invincibility, particularly when they are having a manic episode?"

Prescription Medication and Sometimes Illegal Drug Abuse

I was devastated when, in 1975, I learned about Betsy's overdose on quaaludes. Once admitted to Butler Hospital at Brown University in Providence, Rhode Island, she was diagnosed with the disorder. Apparently, she had used drugs to sedate herself from the manic phases and venomous thoughts she could not stop. Although smoking marijuana and hashish was common in the two states (Pennsylvania and Massachusetts) we lived in during our teens, Betsy graduated to legally prescribed medications.

Her abuse of prescription medications and occasional use of illegal drugs evolved over many years, and because most of her inappropriate behavior was due to abuse of legally prescribed medications, it was an effortless way for her to stay high (i.e., she sought and received painkillers and sleep medications).

After my parents passed away and I became the payee for her Social Security Disability checks, I received all her Medicare and prescription lists and out-of-pocket bills. Year, after year, after year, she was on a great variety of medications, which would change on a frequent basis. I thought to myself, "Eventually, having all these drugs in her system might destroy her organs." One example is her abuse of laxatives, which she started to use because other medications caused constipation, and which led to her inability to control her bowel movements. I know about this in detail because on numerous occasions she would ask me to buy and mail her laxatives. I also remember horrible times with this condition, including an accident she had in a rental car, which my husband had to clean up. Fortunately, she eventually got off laxatives.

Another horrible and embarrassing incident occurred when Betsy and I were shopping for clothes at the Goodwill store in Nanuet, New York. We entered the store, and she immediately ran to the back to the bathroom and shouted, "I am going to go in my pants!" I remember that a key was needed, so I walked very fast to the front desk to get it, and by the time I made it to the back of the store, she had peed all over the floor. I unlocked the bathroom door and proceeded back to the front desk to ask for some paper to clean up the floor. As I recall, at the time she was hooked on laxatives and could not control her bowel movements or urination.

Whenever she had an embarrassing physical accident, I never raised my voice and quietly and quickly cleaned up the mess. I always knew that she was embarrassed and became more accepting of each incident because most of the time she apologized to me.

When Betsy had control of her medications (i.e., the doses were not distributed by pharmacy staff), according to my mother, Betsy went on occasion to a hospital in a toxic state because she had taken more than the required dosage because she was depressed and wanted to end her life. Since 1987, I cannot count the number of times she changed psychiatrists. According to my mother, she "changed shrinks when she could no longer get the medications she desired."

During her stays at numerous hospitals in several states (Florida, Georgia, Massachusetts, New Jersey, New York,

Virginia), where her actions were strictly monitored, she became more stable and would sometimes admit that she was a prescription medication abuser, which caused most of her problems. I wished and prayed that someday she would have the strength to stay on her medications and give the different combinations time to work instead of getting frustrated and then asking for a medication change.

The letter on the next few pages begins with her wants and needs and what she was doing to help herself; it progresses to her main focus—her medication.

Dear Diary,

I really would appreciate a good sound system esp. for the Rolling Stones and Motown. It works well for having fun. I'll have to see how much room and freedom I have. I got a little coffee maker + cooler inside of a cooler, a bookcase would be nice, Reebox + Calvins. I feel good now but have allergies pretty often and cannot take stuff for it. I do a good walk + swim but I am still better off with the bike + weights. I have middle age spread. My boobs + waist are gross. I don't even have a reading lamp in my room now and over the years only 2 or 3 so-so ones from the apartments have survived. at least I have nice den furniture + crafts. My bed + comforters are great. Remind mom a few comforters + good sheets + feather pillows arrive. Helps me to relax.

Maybe a lake will be fun. I caught bish here in St. Pete w/kids, It's fun.

you will notice that as I get better
I can channel into writing, creativity,
reading, exercise, excursions instead
of upset impulsive phone calls. You can
send me cute things (your taste in
clothes is the best — navy shorts + top 😖)
and send cards becuz I save them.
        I see a great psychiatrist 3-4 x
week. In case you are curious for
your NAM, speak ups I take
        Depakote 500   3 x day
        Klonopin 1 mg   4 x day
        Theragram   1 x day
        Chloral Hydrate   2 hs (hour of sleep)
        (Birth c. Pill) and Paxil - antidep.'
        I see a psychiatrist nurse 1x week at
9 am. She's very smart and explains the
meds and this new antidepressant. She's
really pissed because it's so noisy + messy
There's garbage and homosexuality —
ultimately I have been so stressed
out I'm sleeping only 6 hrs. on
NARCOTICS, on NARCOTICS — chloral
hydrate. It'll balance out today when
I get back on the Klonopin — see

Another trait of those suffering from bipolar disorder is deciding not to take the medications prescribed to them. I've spoken with other people who have mentally ill relatives and who have observed or were told about the same behavior—when the person is feeling very good, they decide that they do not need to take their medication(s).

My sister grew dependent on doctor-prescribed medications. Lithium stabilized her moods, and tranquilizers helped her to sleep; later she took heart and thyroid medications. The other tragedy is that, on the occasions when the doctors took her off all medication to clean her system, she would find a way to obtain more painkillers. In addition, after so many years of being on lithium, this medication became toxic to her system, and she could no longer take the drug that kept her stable for nine years. Discontinuing this drug was unfortunate for Betsy, because during her nine-year "calm" time, between 1975 and 1984, lithium was a miracle medication.

My sister used to refer to her state of mind as the "Black Pit" and told me that she could handle the Black Pit because, as horrible as it was, it was much better than a manic phase.

Sometimes it's hard to draw the line between drug abuse and the prescribed medication.

For thirty-five years, my sister moved around the country, while in school she lived in Massachusetts, Rhode Island, Connecticut, Arizona, Florida, World Campus Afloat, Pennsylvania, and thereafter in New Jersey, Florida, and New York, from town to town and county to county. She also moved from one ACLF to another ACLF, from psychiatric hospital to psychiatric hospital, and in and out of general hospitals for medical reasons. I believe all that moving from place to place is what eventually took a toll on her body, stamina, and passion for life. I observed the changes in person, on the phone, in letters, and in conversations with medical professionals. Betsy's life experience became mine, because I allowed myself to be so involved. During and after phone calls and visits, I cried and was despondent, but I always pulled myself together, because I knew that I would be of no help to her if I were incapacitated.

I wondered sometimes if the medications "fried" her brain and slowly killed all her useful brain cells. Having dealt with people who have died from cancer, I know that sometimes the medication and chemotherapy are more toxic than the illness and may kill the patient before the cancer does. Betsy's medications changed frequently, partly because of the contraindications of the different medications combined, which resulted in worse feelings and behavior. Negative physical side effects can also be very debilitating and cause further frustration and depression. This is especially true when an individual is using prescription medications, over-the-counter medications, and street drugs.

In summary, I continually wondered how many years she would be able to cope with her illness and worried about what would become of her.

I have included a number of letters that she wrote to me in which she reflected on her misuse of drugs.

Dear Lindsey,

I wrote! I got some pretty stationary. I colored my hair but maybe too much. Mom's due over today for the doctor's appt's and a few errands. Thank god she does my better laundry too or it comes out so bleach or not at all. I made 4 necklaces and have 8 creative and want to do 3 or 4 × more track - minister, I forgot my lists, on the calendar it says you've cared more busy than any friend ever could. Yea, Lindsey Thank you for your compassion.

I dislike everyone here except some of the staff. You walk on the floors + bell it's so grimy. I feel so up and down about what I can give from here. I like the money goodies and special treat most I get because there true and my clothes, I haven't gotten high since Jan. so I get a pretty soon and so, so shopping. I finally bought a watch but I don't know if it's water proof when I swim I haven't gotten high I mean no joke, I didn't drink anyway but I like try the vodka and to meds. It's water under the bridge, again I went writing, reading + ways to keep to work on in my room because I stay in my room I don't get

Dear Linsey,

I'm enjoying the teas & book you sent. I love my apt. It's so much bigger. I was in the hospital again for medication poisoning — God was I sick! No seizures this time. Please write to me & send me 20.00 if you can. I want us to visit again. My penmanship is poor but I'm trying. I'm working out everyday again + using the tramp. I need to lose weight. The protein powder you got me is excellent! Thanks for thinking of me. Love,
Betsy

Suicide Attempts

There are many reasons people with a mental disorder attempt or commit suicide. Unless the person expresses a desire to die, their loved ones often do not realize the life-threatening danger or have minimal awareness of it. This is another tragic characteristic of someone with bipolar disorder. My sister survived at least three suicide attempts. In the letter below (she originally wrote it by hand; I typed and saved a copy, but lost the original), she described her suicidal thoughts:

> October 1992
>
> Hi,
>
> I love the gorgeous samples and perfume from today. Today I start a new experimental medicine. I have hope but am scared too. The Bal a Versailles is fantastic. Six weeks ago, I got put on Klonopin (for seizures and to relax) and I feel solid like myself and I've slept well since. I exercise and walk daily. I'm not so tan but look good. Need my hair cut and colored (when!!!) It's long now. I look for jobs and walk around the main road A1A and ask. After summer, the $5/hr. opportunities die down but I'm not giving up. I still get pretty severely depressed and don't eat. Linsey please be my helper when mummy or daddy go. Otherwise I'll commit suicide too. I save pills. Help me.
>
> Love, Betsy

Bipolar individuals are strongly advised to not drink alcohol while on their medication, nor should they miss medication doses, because the effects can be toxic and dangerous. In 1988, an excuse Betsy used for becoming suicidal was that one of the medications she was taking, Prozac, made her suicidal and aggressive. This may not have actually been an excuse, because I have read that Prozac has made some people suicidal.

Over the years, my parents and I managed to cope as best as we could and go on with our lives, especially after one of Betsy's suicide attempts. My parents were voracious readers, which was an escape from the agony of my sister's illness. My mother also told me to find an empty box, find a white piece of paper, write my negative and depressing thoughts on it, fold up the paper, put it in the box, close the box, and put it in the corner of a closet, never to think about it again. Sometimes this strategy worked.

We also did our utmost to not allow her illness to prevent us from living and loving our lives. Life is not fair, is often tragic, and has many winding roads and hills to climb, but my sister's hills were the steepest. I climbed many hills with her and was always grateful when she survived her suicide attempts. Beginning in 1984, when I became more involved in her life, and thereafter, I just put one foot in front of the other and jogged or walked down the road. I have been saying to myself for years, "Just put one foot in front of the other and keep moving."

Grandiosity

Betsy always had extravagant ideas and needs, which is another characteristic of bipolar disorder. She always wanted the best of everything and spent money as if it grew on a tree, buying exotic perfume, new clothes, new shoes, coats, designer sheets, jewelry, sessions at the tanning salon, etcetera, and she expected me, my parents, her ex-husbands, or her friend Drew (she wrote about him in some of her letters) to pay for everything.

Grandiose, unrealistic thinking and a desire for things one cannot afford appears to be very common among the bipolar population. Sometimes, I surmised that if she'd had enough of her own money and no financial worries, she would have liked herself better. Maybe then, if her life had been less restrictive regarding material needs, she might not have mishandled her medication. Over the years I realized that even if she had been abundantly wealthy, she would not have been able to control her spending.

I previously mentioned a cab driver calling me to pay for Betsy's cab fare, which was not the only time this happened. Another time, a cab driver called me and asked me to give him my credit card number to pay for my sister's cab. I demanded to speak with her, at which point she verified that she owed him the money, he was in a hurry, and I needed to pay him. I reluctantly approved the release of the money, at which point she emphasized that she needed more money to buy clothes.

Another aspect of Betsy's grandiosity was that she would brag to others about how smart she was because she completed a master's degree in psychiatric social work from the University of Pennsylvania and received almost-perfect scores on all her college entrance tests, and would assert that she was smarter and better than the social worker who was running the group counseling sessions that she attended. This is partially true, because one of the counselors at the hospital told me that Betsy did a very good job running the group counseling meetings.

My mother spent her entire Social Security check on Betsy's needs, and each month my husband and I supplemented her disability income. A classic example of Betsy's grandiosity: At a department store she could spend hundreds of dollars in five minutes, and she would always order the most expensive meal on the menu, with several appetizers. When she moved into Evergreen Court in Spring Valley, New York, in 2008, I deposited $500 into her resident account. Less than a week later, she called and said she needed more money because she had spent every cent at Target for things she needed for her room.

Betsy was luckier than many mentally ill people because, in addition to the Social Security disability check she received, beginning in 1989, she also received an additional stipend from the State of New York. Due to Betsy's grandiose expectations, the $200 per month that remained after I paid her housing and cable bills wasn't enough to cover her toiletries, luxuries, and other incidentals. For many years, my mother and I would send her care packages, always by priority mail, because she pressured us to do so. I did not mind spending money on her, but I disliked the pressure she put on me. A mentally healthy person could create and live on a budget if needed, but Betsy expected others to continuously help her.

One of the ways the Social Security system works is that if they find out that the recipient has received funds from any other sources, the recipient will have to pay back the money.

After my father passed away, Betsy and I each received a military service check for $5,000. The money went into her bank account, and when it was audited by Social Security staff, I had to meet with them and reimburse them.

Their Own Worst Enemy / Alienation from Loved Ones

My sister was her own worst enemy. Because of her manic highs and terrible lows, and because her jumbled, confused, erratic, bizarre, chronic, and difficult-to-deal-with behaviors were so awful at times, she thought she had no choice but to attempt suicide. I believe that this is a classic example of being your own worst enemy. My assessment is that during these times she was experiencing "the black hole" she had described, from which she felt there was no escape until her mood stabilized.

Depression would overcome her, as did anger and frustration about a state of being she could not control. She probably hated herself for this; she may have felt this way and may have felt these dark emotions because many people she met were not suffering the way she was. However, her actions hurt the ones closest to her. Despite all the love and care that my mother and I gave her, she had a pervasive feeling of loneliness. She also wrote mean comments about my father even though he continually ensured that she was taken care of. In a notecard Betsy sent me, she wrote many negative comments about our father, which, of course, upset me.

Dear Linse,

Isn't this pretty stationary? Thankyou so much for your consideration + generosity. I guess it's daddy ... but how does he expect me to get toothpaste, shampoo, why do I have to depend on Drew? I mean it's really nice that he cares but when he calls he's so verbally abusive and sarcastic. His family has <u>tons</u> of money. Oh get this - his oldest sister's 5th husband is Bi Polar but he's an aeronautical engineer + she's a dentist. Well she decided to come home for 6 months for a break 'cuz they were both doing alot of grass. Well, mummy's not even sure I can come home for X-mas. What do they think I am, an axe

Linsey Willis

As noted previously, my sister's feelings about my father affected their relationship for many years until his passing.

I keep referring to the Black Hole because Betsy often told me that during her mood swings, she would feel as though she was inside a black hole from which she could not escape. The feelings of despair and pain caused her to display much vile, angry behavior. But this behavior just caused her alienation from others. For example, I happened to find out she once accidentally recorded a conversation with a childhood friend of hers, Drew, from Upper Saint Clair Township in Pennsylvania. He was a schizophrenic, was on medication that greatly helped him, and he was able to hold down a job as a welder. In that conversation, which I overheard, she invited Drew to stay at my apartment for a few weeks. When I casually mentioned it to her, she threw the iron at me, screamed at me, and called me a lesbian FBI agent. Although Drew was not a stranger to me, the fact that she invited him to stay at my apartment without asking me first was inappropriate behavior.

Another time, she called our father a freak, went after him with a shoe, and began to hit him. On another occasion, she told me she hoped that I and my husband would get killed in a car accident, and said she was going to hire someone to kill my father because then she and our mother could get all his money. The serious problem this presents is that the listener will have difficulty distinguishing between reality and fantasy. This may result in an overprotectiveness of oneself and could cause the listener to withdraw from the ill person.

When you are dealing with a person afflicted with bipolar

illness, whose moods may change every few days or hours, remember that their vile words are just words, and in the big scheme of their mental illness, they may be meaningless. They do not remember what they have said and may not understand why you are responding differently to them. Being the recipient of Betsy's vile words would alienate me for a period of time. However, when I would remind her of the vile words she said to me, she would have no recollection. She would, however, sometimes apologize to me over the phone or in one of her letters.

Bipolar individuals often forget what they said or did and do feel great remorse or guilt over what happened. There were times that I thought Betsy had some sociopathic tendencies because of her absence of remorse, guilt, or shame, but when she did apologize, I was elated. Sadly, there were several times over the years when I did not speak to my sister for a month or so because I was so upset over an incident. My avoiding contact with her by not answering the phone or not returning calls was alienation she had caused. I often felt so guilty that I overcompensated and let her take advantage of me when she was in her manic state. As debilitating as was for me at the time, I never gave up on her and was there for her.

Betsy was evicted from her living quarters on more than six occasions during the 1990s for a variety of reasons. Each time, she blamed someone else or other tenants. However, during most incidents, I failed to remember that she was seriously ill and blaming others was a defense mechanism.

I vividly remember the following events:

- Betsy's apartment had been broken into, and because of this, she called the police and was then taken to the hospital. I do not know if her apartment had actually been broken into, but I do know that she went to the hospital after the police came to her apartment.

- The police arrived at her apartment after she shoplifted, which caused a disturbance for the residents. I know that this incident is true because the apartment manager called my parents after she was arrested. She denied that she had done anything wrong.

- She overdosed on one of her medications and was wandering around the apartment building and stole someone's outside plants. This story is accurate because the apartment manager called my parents. Then Betsy was taken to the hospital.

- Betsy was asked to move out of an ACLF she lived in in Florida because she had been taking food out of the facility to give to the man she was dating, who had been fired from his job and had no money for food. This is a true story, although she denied what the facility manager told my parents. After much discussion, they allowed her to stay.

Betsy's multiple evictions and my involvement in just about every occurrence contributed to my feeling, at times, that I did not want anything else to do with her. But neither my parents nor I abandoned her.

Over the years she also alienated most of the friends she had met along the way. She would opine to me that she was no longer associating with these new friends or neighbors because they were selfish, stupid, dirty, religious freaks, etcetera. Her verbal abuse of people and the putting down of others were probably some of the main reasons she lost friends. Why should people take abuse, particularly from someone they had just met? There are occasions when we take abuse from people at work and in social situations though we don't feel we deserve to, especially when it is a mentally ill person. Many people have negative thoughts about mentally ill people and feel very uncomfortable around them.

Family members often have to find a way of coping with the anger and vile remarks as a way to survive manic or depressed episodes, but this is not an easy nor pleasant state of mind to be forced into on an ongoing basis. However, if you are compassionate enough and do not have any plans to abandon them, God forbid, you will have to store their remarks in a quiet place in the back of your head and try to forgive and forget.

Betsy always hurt the ones who loved her the most, and she undoubtedly loved us. I have met families who had been doing it for over thirty years and others who abandoned their formerly loved one years before! As I have stated, I believe Betsy hated herself for her diagnosis, what her illness had done to her and the family, and what she could not be. She had such potential.

In the late 1990s, Betsy was sent to a dual-diagnosis treatment program that was much better than the state facilities, local hospitals, or the centers where she had to go, on occasion, once she had used up all her allowed stays in the regular hospitals. Not only was she in the appropriate place for her, but according to my mother and her, it was also very plush and private. Nonetheless, she checked herself out because she didn't like the detoxifying process and insisted she couldn't go without any medications. With each stay in a facility she ended up disliking the people there and feared ever having to go back. This is another example of the alienation she caused.

Another incident involved her self-admittance to a hospital because she claimed that she had been beaten up by someone at her place of residence. The hospital staff looked for evidence of bruises but found none. At the time I felt strongly that she may have caused someone to strike her, if, in fact, they did. My other thought was that she used having been hurt and beaten as an excuse to get painkillers.

In the late 1990s, Betsy was admitted to a another supposedly long-term dual-diagnosis treatment program on the west coast of Florida. At the end of a three-month period—during which time she was feeling great, making new friends, and feeling hopeful—they temporarily sent her to a retirement home until they could find an appropriate ACLF. Even though a court order placed her in this program due to her numerous evictions and shoplifting charges, when her paid hospital days were exhausted, she was immediately discharged and moved to another facility. Then, less than one month later, she was caught trying to steal additional medication from the facility.

The mental health system seems designed to get mentally ill people well enough so they can be released back into the community, but not to help them for the long term, because this costs money. How can anyone get even partially stable with this pattern? The system also appears to not be designed to get dual-diagnosis patients permanently off the drugs they abuse. The next paragraph is about one such story.

Soon after my sister had been admitted to the aforementioned dual-diagnosis treatment program, she was again hopeless; she continually complained about how terrible the facility was, that the other mentally ill people were worse off than she, and that the food was terrible. Each time she was released from a psychiatric hospital, her system was cleaned out, and she was better and more hopeful about her life, despite the fact that her life was a roller coaster.

Sometimes the merry-go-round went fast and other times very slowly, and I was a regular passenger and could not get off it. Also, my sister's sad life was a merry-go-round, and during the early years of her illness, she hoped she would get better. Her merry-go-round included self-medicating, running out of money, stealing from housemates, exploding into a manic or depressed phase, exhibiting sexual promiscuity, and attempting suicide.

As I stated earlier, my dear mother, who spent an inordinate amount of time with my sister during the early years of her illness, noted that Betsy seemed to be on her best behavior while hospitalized. But once released from the hospital, she had to face loneliness and the stark reality of her existence, and as a result, would punish herself and others around her.

Back to the "own worst enemy" topic: My sister was her own worst enemy, because during her depressed states, she was angry and verbally abusive to boyfriends, one of her husbands, friends, and family, and when she was manic, she was out of control.

In summary, we grew to understand that she would never have a "normal" life, but we hoped and prayed that someday she would stop abusing herself, gain some strength to deal more realistically with her illness, work harder to gain some semblance of order, and find some peace in her life.

Somewhere around 1948, the Mills Brothers sang, "You always hurt the one you love, the one you shouldn't hurt at all. You always take the sweetest rose and crush it till the petals fall."

Master Manipulator

My sister had a manipulative and dominant personality. She was successful in dominating me when we were growing up. Most of the time, I allowed her to have things her way. She was my older sister, and I looked up to her. Often it was difficult to distinguish what portion of her manipulative nature and dominance was caused by the illness and what portion was inherent to her true personality. As Betsy attempted to gain some semblance of order in her life, she used other people and did her best to manipulate them to get what she needed. Her manipulation tactics resulted in my parents and me reacting to and jumping to the occasion. Sometimes my sister "cried wolf"—there were times when she would telephone my parents with what they perceived as an almost life-shattering need for food or assistance, and when they arrived to help her, she was perfectly fine. Once again, her manipulation tactics had worked. People close to her rose to the occasion. We loved her and closed our eyes when she behaved abnormally.

Another form of manipulation was when, on many occasions, she verbalized to my mother in a threatening way, "When you and Dad die, I'll kill myself; I'll have no one else." When my mother told me this, I was very sad and scared. In my rationalization I thought that she was just acting, but I really didn't know.

Betsy also always managed to get whatever she wanted from my parents, while I had to painfully beg to get what I wanted—for example, a pair of skis. Her intelligence and ability to manipulate situations enabled her to get what she wanted her entire life. Even though my sister was my dad's favorite, I know that he was greatly saddened by what he considered her wasted life. Moreover, my mother always told me that he loved both of us a great deal. It is so unfair, because he had such lofty expectations for Betsy.

If your mentally ill loved one, child, or sibling tries to manipulate you, let me tell you to make sure than another child is not overlooked, ignored, or marginalized. I know it's hard not to have a favorite child. However, when it is quite obvious that one child is having major problems—such as experimenting with drugs, demonstrating weird behavior, being promiscuous, having weird highs and lows, and being verbally abusive—you should seek help immediately. As a parent, it is so important to ensure that the other son or daughter is not left out of the communication loop. You need to recognize and not ignore the pain that your other child may feel.

Linsey Willis

Need to Be the Center of Attention

Betsy always needed to be the center of attention. Given her constant mental state and emptiness, it's understandable that she focused on herself so much, with what she had to face every morning. Her attention-getting tactics and self-centeredness were difficult to deal with, especially when she would project onto another person. For example, she would often call my mother a selfish bitch. My mother was not the least bit selfish.

Even though I have had a very successful, happy, and healthy career, a wonderful and supportive husband, and many wonderful friends, when I was growing up and after Betsy's illness emerged, she was my parents' main focus. Regardless of her illness, being on the bottom of my parents' priority list wounded what self-esteem I had. I believe I became an overachiever because it was a defense mechanism. Being fully occupied with work, education, exercise, my husband, and friends helped me keep my mind off Betsy, by being busy.

Many times, I surmised that Betsy had to be the center of attention because her needs were so great that being paid attention to made her feel better. In essence, she relied heavily on her lifeline: our parents and me.

Promiscuity, Numerous Boyfriends, and Marriages

When Betsy was eligible to work, she always had a part-time job, in high school and every summer, as well as a boyfriend or several teenagers she was dating. During her teens and until she was diagnosed with a bipolar disorder in 1975 at age nineteen, her life seemed to be incredibly positive, except that she always had to have a man in her life and was promiscuous. She would tell me about a new man she met, that she had slept with him, but then after a few meetings, she did not like him anymore. I view having sex with different men that you hardly know as being promiscuous.

She ended the relationships with two of the best boyfriends: Scott, whom I vividly recall and who wanted to marry her; and the other one, who happened to be from one of the richest and most well-known families in the United States. To protect his privacy, I have omitted his name. However, after she met some of his family members at one of their estates in New Jersey, she ended the relationship. I believe she ended the relationship because she didn't have the confidence to continue it. More than likely, she was intimidated by his wealth and family name. My parents had met him several times and liked him, primarily because they believed he would be good for Betsy.

Another excuse she used to end some of her relationships and marriages was that she said there was something wrong with each man. She also told me that she felt she was not good enough or rich enough for them, but I believe it was because she was afraid they would find out about her illness. She was projecting onto them. I do not know if her first husband or Betsy ended the marriage or whether the other relationships she had were ended by her or the men. I surmise that the men ended the relationships because they could not deal with her disability. It is very difficult, even for family members, to initially cope with the manic-depressive behavior.

According to my sister, over the years, the different medications dulled her sex life. Although people with bipolar disorder are known to be sexually promiscuous, based on what I have read, my sister sometimes told me that she did not enjoy sex or receive pleasure from the act. From my perspective, that was an oxymoron because she usually had sex early in a relationship. The excitement of being with a new man may have increased her hormonal arousal, but that arousal may have quickly diminished if she spent time with the man.

Betsy appeared to have a very good nine-year relationship with Frank, the mentally ill boyfriend who lived at the same assisted living facility, Evergreen Court, in Spring Valley, New York. However, most of her other relationships and her three marriages were much shorter. Betsy and Frank were very supportive of one another. The two of them are in the photo on the next page.

Like many other mentally disabled people, he worked for many years, had a psychotic breakdown, went on permanent disability, got divorced, and then lived with his mother and sister until they determined it would be better if he moved to an ACLF. I spent time with him every time I went to visit Betsy. He provided her with love and stability, for which I was grateful. He was always there for her, and she for him, which I was very happy about. He was a wonderful human being.

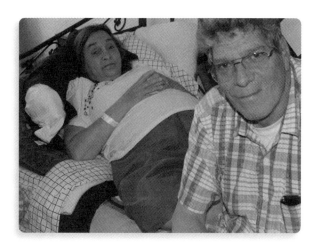

It was tragic that he went to the hospital during the first year of the pandemic and died there, not of COVID-19 but from other ailments he never knew existed. My sister was so devastated because, due to COVID-19 restrictions, she was unable to visit him. The loss of Frank just added to her experiences with losing loved ones. I was so grateful that his sister and mother stayed in touch with her for a short time after his death.

During the nine years Betsy spent with Frank, I was so grateful, felt a sense of peace for her, and hoped that they would be together for the rest of their lives. I was greatly saddened when he passed on. She felt lost. However, I thanked God that she'd had some joy and happiness in her life, all those years with Frank. I thought to myself, "What more tragedy does Betsy have to experience?"

About six months after Frank's death, a fire demolished the facility where Betsy was living. That horrible incident caused so much pain and sorrow. I will never get over the horror of what happened. (See Chapter 9: The Fire and Beginning of the End.)

Easily Agitated—Could Not Accept Criticism

At the flip of a switch, Betsy would move from one stage to another. She would verbally lash out at me if I made a comment about her agitated behavior and what she was doing. For example, she would become impatient while waiting at the checkout counter at Target, and then she would become even more agitated when I asked her to stop or slow down. She had a very low tolerance for anyone correcting or criticizing her, and the stress would cause her to lash out at the individual. She would also become agitated whenever money was involved, because no matter how much I gave her, it was never enough.

Betsy was also very critical of other people and tended to look down on them. I remember when she was still working, she would make disparaging comments about the nurses at the hospitals where she worked. She possessed a master's degree in social work and told me she specialized in psychiatric social work at the University of Pennsylvania. Betsy always thought she knew more than the nurses and had difficulty dealing with the stressful situations that are common at hospitals. Any problems she told me about with her coworkers were always their fault.

There were other times, particularly during holiday dinners, when she would instigate a fight with someone by making a snide remark. When our mother reminded Betsy that she should not drink any alcohol because of the medications she was taking, instead of accepting the advice, she would lash out. She sometimes got up from the table and left the house. Many times when I took her on shopping trips, she would also instigate fights or scream at me in a loud voice. This often happened when I told her that there were enough items in the shopping cart and that we had exceeded the budget.

On some occasions, the stressful situations, which she often caused, resulted in her self-admittance to the hospital. She would have the staff who worked at the reception desk at Evergreen Court, Spring Valley, New York, call an ambulance. While married to her second husband (whose name I do not recall because I never met him) in 1990, she was stable for about one year. But when the relationship started to crumble, she became manic or depressed. At one point she was in an auto accident, wrecked the car but was not injured, and went back into the hospital. As noted previously, she used the hospital as a place to escape, as well as a place to get stabilized. Overall, the pattern was repeated many times over the years. We were all sad whenever she was admitted to a psychiatric hospital but were grateful that she had the medical coverage for even a limited period of time. We were also grateful that her basic safety and security needs were being taken care of while hospitalized.

Another key stressor for Betsy was her ongoing fear of what would happen to her when my parents died. My parents and I always told her that she would be taken care of. I reinforced this by telling her I would always be there for her, no matter what!

Nonfulfillment of Plans

My sister was not able to make or complete any plans which was attributed to her continual highs, lows, and racing mind. The only times she ever seemed to have a plan in her life were when she had a boyfriend, during which time she made plans to set up housekeeping with him. In an academic setting, she was secure and was able to burn off her manic energy through her studies. She always completed her assignments on time. All through college, she maintained a 4.0 GPA, had great writing abilities, analytical and synthesis skills, and was good at dealing with people, particularly outside of family members.

After about twelve years working in the social work profession, she reached a point where the illness took control of her life, and she could no longer work in a stress-filled profession. Her illness caused her too much stress and anxiety. This was understandable; she was having great difficulty dealing with herself, let alone other people and their issues.

A letter she wrote to me about her life plans was intertwined with comments about her mood swings and desire to work part time. As with all her letters, this one is particularly heart wrenching.

Dear Linsey & Frank,

I am very sad and in pain because after the manic episode is the dull depression. But! I can foresee bringing more good things into my life this time and having more say so about goal things happening to me. We are the masters of our own fate. I do feel ready to work part time and even I wonder if I'll ever get good help anymore; but, the nurses say I'm doing better and better each day. Drew calls often — he's really hung up on going back to night school but his aspirations are always unrealistic. Right now he has a decent job & no expenses.

Boy, I wish I had a card or a plant or flowers from you. Mom brought pj's, books & good cheer. I still love my

apartment and the strange social
life at the pool. I love the
tanning salon too. I'm lying
to buy some shoes, 2 outfits
wax my eyebrows, maybe get a
kitty & start working out (2 hrs
day!) For the 8th time I had
PMS then came to the hospital
& got my period. I need a
good endocrinologist. I'm
sleepy + feel full from
spaghetti. I better not gain an
ounce — I'm 120 now.

        Love Betsy
        Write / Call!

Once she applied for and received Social Security Disability benefits, any grand plans she might have previously had ceased. Fortunately, her plans to have her teeth fixed were taken care of by our father. She used to have large, square, beautiful, white, shiny, and almost perfect teeth, but being on medications for so many years ruined them. Based on what she told me, her teeth were starting to deteriorate, chip, and loosen in her mouth.

She stopped planning for her future because of her fear of failure, mood swings, and decreasing lack of confidence and self-esteem. Our mother then handled all the long-term plans for Betsy. After the deaths of our parents in 2006 and 2007, and until Betsy's death on September 4, 2022, Frank, my dear supporting husband, and I took care of Betsy's very short-term plans. A large part of being there for someone all the time is showing up, which sometimes requires quick adjustments and arrangements. As her illness worsened, Betsy's life plans basically consisted of making sure she had a boyfriend and somewhere to live.

Betsy wrote the following letter to me, full of hope about one of the psychiatric hospitals to which she was admitted.

Dr's Ideas: "Modification of my
internal responses to stress is where
the $ is at!" + this psychiatrist
says for me: "no redemption
through medication." he wants me
to use inner resources more so
one of the things I'm doing is
writing + reading more.

a'right so, the 'medical' doctor
put on the treatment plan for
me to keep learning about symptoms
of active hepatitis C and hypo-
thyroidism – neither of which is
there a cure for but I really
do feel fine. I have to be
careful about germs, though.

I like to keep busy +
exercise, especially walking.
Mom sent me the book
Angels + Demons which is going

I wanted to tell you about my treatment plan – it's psychiatric & medical goals; let me give you some examples: Well it's so long but the 2 main ones are:

"Betsy will maintain behavioral control & stable mood when confronted w/ daily stressors, to be confirmed by her own report and by staff observations."

"Betsy will report report that her mania or hypomania is at a level where she can function through the day without agitation, intrusiveness on others, or disturbed thought processes to be confirmed by her own + staff report."

Other ideas on my treatment plan are about post – traumatic stress disorder: being able to discuss things w/ specific staff + handling feelings + knowing how the past effects currents thoughts + behavior. That's ALOT!!

I'm trying to keep busy until medication time – I really feel like I need some + it'll help me concentrate better.

I've got alot of nice cosmetics + clothes now from the

SHOCK TREATMENTS 04

Overview

One of many great tragedies of my sister's life was the number of shock treatment sessions she experienced. The last series may have helped her the most, because a year or so before her death, one of the doctors told me she had not had a psychiatric episode for over six years. I really don't know whether that was true, and it is difficult to ascertain how it affected her intellectual personality.

Sometime between 2012 and 2015, I had planned to visit Betsy in Spring Valley, New York, and stopped to visit my friends Alan and Brenda. On this trip Brenda and I decided that I would go with her to Atlantic City for a few days, and then she would drop me off at the car rental facility at the Newark airport. I have included my visit with Brenda to illustrate another example of how my life was intertwined with Betsy's life. We decided that I should visit Betsy after my visit with them, because I would have some relaxation and fun after my visit with Betsy. Each time I visited Betsy, Murphy's Law—which is that anything that can go wrong will go wrong—was enacted through no fault of my own.

For this particular trip, the stress began when I arrived in Newark. Betsy called me and was in a very manic and agitated state. She asked me to stop by the Nanuet mall and buy her some designer sheets that she had read about, as well as some other items. She was talking very fast and was being aggressive. On or before our return from Atlantic City, and before I arrived at the rental car counter, I received the first call from Betsy, who was in a psychiatric hospital in Rockland County, New York. I do not recall which one, but I knew that I would have to change hotels and would be charged for not giving enough notice, because the hotel was quite a distance from where she lived in Spring Valley. On a map, Spring Valley and Nanuet are right next to each other, but the hotel I changed to was several miles away. I usually stayed at the Hampton Inn on Route 59 in Nanuet, New York. I did not like driving in New York and wanted to be as close to the hospital as possible. However, I was not looking forward to having to visit her in a hospital during the few days I was going to be there.

Betsy was having a very bad manic episode, and she told me that she would be having shock treatments while she was there. My heart skipped a beat and of course I was worried. I had never been with her at a hospital during shock treatments. I told her I would see her soon, hung up the phone, and then proceeded to the rental car counter, at which point I was advised that there was no car reservation in my name for that weekend but rather for the following weekend, which was not what I was told or had on my paperwork. The person at the desk appeared to be a new hire and was not sure of what to do. The lines were fairly long, so the other representatives could not help the newly hired employee or me. My stress level rose when I was told that they had few cars, only larger cars were available, and the price would be more than I had expected. I was already very upset about where Betsy was and because I had not budgeted a few hundred dollars more for a rental car for three to four days at the last minute and because Betsy had already called me several times, asking me to bring her clothes and other items to the hospital and as soon as possible. Betsy also talked about what she would be going through. Tears formed in my eyes, my heart started beating faster, and my patience was diminishing, so I made a quick decision to immediately return to Florida.

I left the counter, got on the train, and returned to the airport terminal. Being used to the greed of the airlines, I knew there would be a change fee but not what I was told I had to pay. The change fee cost me almost $1,000 because it was last-minute. I was so upset that I did not care. My mental health was far more important than money. After proceeding through security, I spent the next few hours in a wine bar in the airport, called the staff at Evergreen Court to tell them I would not be coming to see Betsy, called my husband, then drowned myself in wine and cheese.

The staff person I spoke to was very upset that I would not be visiting Betsy at the hospital and pleaded with me to change my mind, at which point I told her it was too late. When I returned home, I did not experience a reflective moment, because I was too upset and unable to wrap my mind around Betsy being in another psychiatric hospital and in the process of having shock treatments. Even the calmest of caretakers have moments of stress, causing them to become quite depressed.

When I returned home, I was still so upset that I did not speak to Betsy for a few weeks. One reason was I did not feel I could mentally handle hearing about what she went through. She was very upset that I did not visit her, but we forgave each other.

The letters on the following pages describe Betsy's past experience with shock treatments.

Dear Linsey,

I need to write to you ASAP as I begin shock treatments tomorrow) so I'll have bad memory & confusion. It's going to take a long time (1 month). Please write, call & esp. send me flowers — I'll need so much support now.

Now, as for you I don't like that you get so sad and worried. Remember to always count your blessings and I

Insist you go see Dr.
Abbey Strauss — he's more
fabulous than Friedenthal.
Not a psychologist! Be honest,
and compassionate give
yourself and each other
space, rest, luxuries. If
you feel vulnerable or fear-
ful it can tell you what's
deeply important to you.
Be open, flow, be direct.
Don't get anxious about what
other people think. Have a

warm bath, a run, a swim,
an ativan — you deserve to
live HAPPILY with Frank
because he's great! The
light you are seeking is inside. The Light is life, is
love, is you. There are
only two emotions — love
or fear. Seek love — it's
the infinite. I LOVE you

Betsy

Dear Linsey,

Thankyou for thinking of me + sending a letter. I know you care deeply + also thankyou for stationary. I sure would like some **beau-tiful stationary** and 12.⁻ to get something special. Send it all Priority Mail if you can. I sure also need a **small perfume**. My musk is missing 😞. I'm listening to Whitney Houston - she's beautiful. How's your family of cats and Frank? I sure have been manic even with meds +

shock treatments. Oh I'm so
defeated and sad sometimes.
But I try to keep it together
and I _do_ take your advice.
Send me some clothes (size 8)
I'm really low. I'll be here
2 or 3 more weeks. Try to
write more. I gotta stop now
because some of the details are
awfully sad : med's, med's, shock
treatments. I'll be doing better
soon...

     Love Betsy

   Try to send clothes, please

TWENTY-ONE MORE YEARS: 2001 TO 2022

Overview

As you can see from the its title, many years are covered in this chapter. A great deal took place during those years, a time when I did not do much writing, for a variety of reasons. They included the September 11 bombing of the World Trade Center, my husband and I moving to a new home in the same city, a period of estrangement from my father, the early retirement of my husband, and the fact that in 2003 I suffered a debilitating car accident, which took me three years to recover from.

These years were fraught with many significant and tragic events in Betsy's life. In this chapter I do my best to include as many of the events as possible, particularly the most unusual, interesting, shocking, debilitating, hopeful, and then dreadful.

Primary Caregiver for Betsy

By 2001, I felt so sad for my parents, because they had been Betsy's caregivers and support system for more than twenty-five years. They retired to Florida in 1987, and by 2001 they had become almost-full-time caregivers. For many years we hoped, and hoped, and hoped that Betsy's life would improve, that she would stop abusing herself and being so self-destructive, eventually find a permanent residence, and start working again, even on a part-time basis. We were not facing reality, which was partially due to our naivete about bipolar disorder, since there is no cure. It was a painful love that we had for Betsy.

Nevertheless, by 2001 we had all learned to be more supportive, better listeners, and less judgmental, and like alcoholics practicing the Twelve Steps, we took one day at a time. Before my parents passed away in 2006 and 2007, I promised to never, ever, ever forsake Betsy, no matter what occurred.

During the last few days of his life, I asked my father if he had any regrets. He said no and that he had finally accepted that Betsy had been born with the illness and did her best to cope with it. However, he shared with me that he regretted that she had used illegal drugs as an escape mechanism. By this time he was being administered morphine and was more relaxed, and he had become more conversational than he had ever been with me in my entire life. It was wonderful that he shared a life review with me and told me tales he had never spoken before. He shared stories about WWII and having been on a navy destroyer. He also read to me letters that he had written to his parents, which they had saved for him. One of the more significant things he expressed was that even though he and my mother had spent over $250,000 of their life savings taking care of Betsy, he had absolutely no regrets and would not have had it any other way. My eyes welled up with tears, and I gave him the biggest hug of my life. Afterward, I wished that we had hugged more during his life.

Moreover, both of our parents were never going to allow Betsy to end up on the streets like millions of mentally ill homeless people living in cities across the United States. Based on my knowledge, mentally ill homeless people who live on the streets do so for variety reasons, but one of the major reasons is that their families have abandoned them because they could not cope with their illnesses. I had a great deal of gratitude that our parents never "washed their hands" of Betsy, and neither did I.

Between 2001 and 2022, on numerous occasions, Betsy was in and out of psychiatric and general hospitals, and I was eternally grateful that she had help and was not homeless. However, had she stayed in Florida, I believe her life would have been far worse, because Florida does not provide resources like the Northeastern states. Florida has no state income tax and is not part of the Medicare expansion system, and it does not have a sufficient number of facilities for the mentally ill. God forbid any of us have to pay part of our taxes to provide for the poor, disabled, and mentally ill members of our society; the following reasons underlie my sarcastic comments:

- No one wants to pay more in taxes.
- We want to pay less in taxes.
- Let the church and family members pay for the disabled and mentally ill, as it is not our responsibility.
- Make sure that wherever they are living, it is not in my backyard (NIMBY).

Since my parents were deceased, I was my sister's only caregiver, other than her long-term boyfriend and a few friends (e.g., Drew). I regularly experienced so many emotions, which included the following:

- *Agony,* when I had to pick her up off the floor after having fallen out of her bed of the hospital because the CNA was busy
- *Fear,* that she might be asked to leave Evergreen Court because of smoking
- *Grief,* because sometimes when I arrived in New York to visit, I found out she had just been sent to the hospital
- *Triumph,* when we had a good time together
- *Elation,* because she loved the new or used clothes I bought for her
- *Frustration,* when she pleaded with me to buy a takeout meal for her boyfriend, Frank, even though she already had plenty of doggy bags for both of them
- *Joy,* when I bought four dozen Dunkin' Donuts doughnuts, a few large pots of coffee, creamer, and sugar for the residents of Evergreen Court, and faces lit up with smiles and verbal thanks
- *Empathy,* when I would chat with the other residents, while visiting Betsy, learn about them and their lives (e.g., how they ended up at an assisted living facility), and occasionally give them a few dollars

- *Happiness,* when Betsy and I enjoyed a nice lunch or dinner because dining out was one of the few joys she had in her life and that we shared together

When Betsy moved from Florida to New Jersey in 2001 with her third husband, Joe, she experienced some of her worst and most traumatic incidents. Some of them included the following:

- feeling very sad and distraught that her husband, Joe, had dispensed with her
- being kicked out of an assisted living facility in New Jersey
- having me help her move to a small town in New Jersey in about 2006 or 2007 because she had broken into a medicine cabinet at her previous living quarters and was evicted
- losing, throwing, or giving away the new suitcases I bought her when she moved to Hackensack
- having her belongings in plastic bags when I picked her up from where she was living
- being arrested for shoplifting and having the police called

Besides being a caregiver, I played many roles: a passive observer, an active participant because I had to deal with or resolve the situation, a mediator, a banker, a disturbance handler, a mover, a negotiator, and a person who "picked up and cleaned the mess." Many of the most challenging, disastrous, sickening, exhausting, and heart-wrenching situations required a significant deal of strength, perseverance, fortitude, and plain guts to deal with them. The examples in the next section cover many years of my sister's disorderly and stressful life.

Move from Florida to New Jersey with New Husband

During 2000 and 2001, my sister was living in Palatka, Florida, and was ordered by the court into a dual-diagnosis treatment center in Boca Raton, Florida. My parents did not tell me that she was moving to Boca Raton because they did not want to cause me stress and they also knew that I would, more than likely, visit her, since I lived in the same city. One evening, my sister called me, told me where she was, and said that she had gotten married to a man named Joe, who was staying in the same treatment facility. She wanted to see me and pleaded with me to take her shopping, and, of course, I made plans to take her to Target. My dear husband, Frank, accompanied me. Betsy was in a manic phase. She tried on one outfit after another and discarded those she did not want, started undressing outside the dressing room, where the clothes racks were, and would not listen to me when I told her to go back into the dressing room.

As we walked outside after purchasing her items, a store security staff person followed us and asked my sister to open her jacket. She did so, and items from the store fell out. I had no idea she had stolen anything, nor did the items have sensors affixed, and I pleaded with man not to arrest her or us. Immediately, I was very worried and scared about what would happen to my husband and me if Target officials decided to arrest us. I told the man at the store about Betsy's mental illness, where she was living, and why. Meanwhile, my husband, who is a quiet and thoughtful person and rarely speaks out unless absolutely necessary, was fuming. His face transmitted his anger. We were fortunate that Betsy was not arrested and we were allowed to leave. Of course, I lashed out at her, and of course she apologized. We dropped her off at the facility and left quickly. Once again, my emotions and thoughts were mixed. I was devastated yet thankful she was not taken to jail, but I was also quite angry, sad, and worried about what would happen next.

My husband, Frank, continued to be very upset. A few days later, Betsy showed up at our home with her new husband, Joe, and they asked to come in and visit. They were on their way to New Jersey to live with his parents until they found a place. Frank did not want them in our house. My husband was still mentally fuming about the recent shoplifting incident. We wished them well, and they drove off. I was happy that she had found a new companion and that she might finally have some stability in her life. I wondered whether they would stay together, and I thought about when I would see her again.

A day or so later, on a late winter evening, I received a call from a state trooper in Virginia. He told me that he found my sister alongside a state highway. She had bags and was just standing there. He asked me when I would be able to pick her up. I was shocked and informed him that I lived in Florida and would not do so. I said that she had recently left Florida with her new husband, and they were on their way to New Jersey.

He was aware of the aforementioned and asked me what I was going to do about her husband, who had dumped her on the side of the road, and where he should take her. I suggested the closest hospital. I do not recall how many days she was at the hospital, but Joe learned where she was and picked her up. A few days later, Betsy called me and told me what happened and said they were living with his parents. This was not the beginning of a great new life for her with her new husband. What happened about a year or so later was sad, shocking, and horrible.

The letter on the following page was written during their first few years of marriage, and in it Betsy references Joe's psychiatric problems.

Dear Linsey + Frank,

Thanks again for reaching out to me. Do you like the pictures? We want to do it again: Tuy + white.

Please pray Joan + Bob (esp. cries(Bob lets us visit on our way down to Boca — Deerfield. We're probably getting a nice apt. in Deerfield.

He's doing his cen today, all day so I get time to myself. Thank god. I really want y us to all meet.

Please don't criticize me to Beth. Joe had a deep psychiatric + misbehavior past, too. But for both of us it's in the past. I promise + I love you guys. Please write, write + call, call #5##0. 8/1 Send a schedule. I have ALL I can do keeping him cheerful + me comfortable well with med. LOT's BEST

Taken to a State Psychiatric Hospital

All was quiet for a while. However, about two years later, I received a call from Joe, who informed me that that he had just dropped Betsy off at a state hospital. He said that he could no longer live with her. He discovered that she was going through his mother's belongings. As a result, his parents did not want her living there and wanted both of them to leave. Given that he suffered from depression and that I knew my sister very well, I was somewhat understanding, but I told him that he had abdicated his responsibility for taking care of his wife. He apparently was not committed to the marriage and was relinquishing his commitment by just leaving his wife at a state hospital. He told me that she needed help because she was always seeking drugs.

I asked for the name of the facility and where it was located in New Jersey. He indicated that he knew where to take her because his brother, who was schizophrenic, lived there

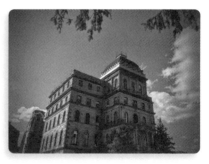

on a permanent basis. I asked him for more information so I could call her, and I hung up the phone.

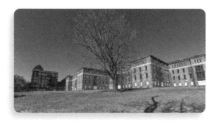

The facility was Greystone Park Psychiatric Hospital in Morris Plains, New Jersey. It was built in 1876 to alleviate over-crowding at the state's only other "lunatic asylum" located in Trenton, New Jersey.[15]

Shortly after Betsy's admission, she sent me a three-page placement-type document. Although I was pleased to have the record, at the same time, I was very sad that her husband took her there, which was the beginning of the end of their marriage. Page 1 of the form follows.

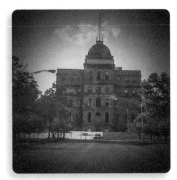

15. https://www.google.com/search?q=greystone+park+psychi-atric+hospital&oq=greystone+park+p&aqs=chrome.0.0i355i-512j46i175i199i512j69i57j0i512l7.7031j0j7&sourceid=chrome& ie=UTF-8.

FYI

Greystone Park Psychiatric Hospital

PLACEMENT TYPE MANUAL & SUMMARY OF NEEDED SKILLS FOR COMMUNITY LIVING -**2003**

PLACEMENT TYPE

*Goes for everywhere
But prices for nre groups
home vary - remember.*

1. Independent Living
Can live without formal supervision on one's own, and does not rely on another or others for aid or support beyond what the average citizen needs. This excludes living in a motel/hotel, mission, or homeless shelter.

2. Rooming House
Can reside without formal supervision in a facility, which provides a safe environment - for Lodging. Meals are not provided.

3. In-Home with Supports
Consumers can reside in their own, or their family's home with multi-disciplinary team availability as needed on a 24 hour basis, i.e.: PACT Support Services.

4. Home with Family
Can reside with relatives who will provide supervision, support and guidance.

5. Residential Intensive Support Services (RIST)
As part of *Redirection II Services* for patients in counties: Passaic, Morris and (Bergen - to be announced) Consumers can reside in their own apartments and supports are available upto 24 hours as needed.
> Passaic - (*RHD*)= Resources for Human Development
> Morris - (*MHA*) = Mental Health Association of Morris County
> Bergen - To Be Announced
> These programs can accommodate *MICA clients* and clients with special medical needs.

6. Family Care (*Essex county*)
Consumers can live in a private home or apartment under the supervision of *a Division of Mental Health Services* provider agency. The agency provides consultation and mental health services to the client based on a Services Agreement. General supervision, support, guidance and some ADL Training may be provided by the Family Care Provider.

7. Boarding Home
Can reside in a facility, which provides a safe environment for lodging and meals, which also provides limited supervision and assistance to clients.

8. Supported Boarding Home (*Class -C*)
Can reside in a licensed (*Class C*) Boarding Home, supplemented by supportive mental health services including,, but not limited to, on-site services and activities to enhance daily living.

The two other pages were as detailed, if not more so. The only positive emotion I had after having read each page was that there were many different types of facilities and services for the mentally ill, and I knew she would be safe there.

I communicated with Betsy frequently while she was at Greystone. The letter below describes her plans for my visit.

so we don't have to plan much. I
really don't know my way around,
There's a great pizza place very close
by that would be fun + it can, not
hang out in my room a little and
walk the grounds alot, ok?
   alright so I'll insert a notecard with my phone numbers and
the nursing station extention number.
   See you. I love you.
      can't wait!
         Love,
         Betsy
Thanks so much for coming ♡

I went to visit my friend Brenda before my visit to Betsy. Brenda offered to go with me. Upon our arrival at the facility, Betsy came to the door, was apparently in a manic phase, and was also very upset. However, I was not allowed to visit her and was not told the reason why. I assumed it was because she was very manic. She was pounding on the window and raising her voice. I told her I would be in touch with her, was in tears, and thought, "How much worse will it get?" Brenda was very consoling.

During the approximately two years Betsy lived at Greystone, Joe visited her frequently. As I recall, he was hopeful that she would get better and they could be together again. But it never happened.

On the following pages is a letter Betsy wrote to me while at Greystone.

Dear Frank + Linse,

Please call me at (973) 347-5100 Room # 145. It is snowing like crazy up here. W/out a phone card I can't call you. Please don't unload alot of dirt on Joe about my past. He had a heavy past, too but since he comes from a big family I think there's more support. We are very lucky + much happier being together + helping each other. My doctor suspects some cancer on the thyroid gland but he promises it can be completely removed. Joe's parents have helped us out financially tremendously. I have written to Joan + Bob that we'd like to visit them on the way back down to Florida for a few days. I am paranoid + tired + get B-12 shots + the nebulizer treatments 1x week. Daddy makes such a big deal about it but look how

young + hit me and I barely smoke
cigs anymore. Even coffee makes me
very hyper. Anyway I have a great doctor.

Listen, please forgive my actions
and know that I love you very
much. Joe is really the first
man I've fallen in love with
where I have the patience to
stick with the hard work + commitment a marriage requires. He is extremely
intelligent but sometimes a handful because
of his temperament.

Another letter Betsy wrote while she was at Greystone
provides a glimpse of what life is like in a psychiatric hospital.
One of the things I always noticed about Betsy's letters was
the variation in her handwriting. There were times when her
handwriting was neat, she did not just write one very long paragraph, and she did not change from one topic to another. These
letters were written when she was stabilized and doing well. The
following letter includes descriptions of the meds she was taking,
her physical condition, and details about her belongings. She
also describes some of the staff, residents, and her roommate,
much of which is criticism.

During this time, her estranged husband, Joe, was still visiting her. Reading the letter carefully, you can learn something
about the life of a very intelligent person living in a psychiatric
hospital.

One of the more interesting sections of the letter is about her friend Drew from Upper Saint Clair High School, whom I wrote about earlier in this book. He was participating in a double-blind study for a new medication for schizophrenia. They kept in touch most of their lives, even during all of Betsy's moves. Finally, I found comfort in the fact that she was doing better, that she bothered to wish my husband, Frank, a happy Father's Day, and that she ended the letter with "I love you!"

June 21

Dear Linsey + Frank,

By the way Frank - Happy belated Father's Day! So this is the first day of summer but it's been summer for you for months now, right?

As you know I'm on the fast-track ultra-nice unit. I am not ready to get discharged. I'm still manic-y + the change was physically + emotionally a toll. But now we have lots of storage space space, maids, laundry that not's locked up or that you have to sign up for.

On Sunday a nice guy here gave me his phone card w/ 7.00 left on it for 3.00 and I tried your home number but it said fax machine or no one home. I've got alot of stuff to work out : ear surgery, back on hormones, getting all the groups + privileges. I want a money slip for patient's accounts to go out on a pass with Joe + also to have money here for the GPA (greystone patient association) which is the huge house used as a consignment store. One whole room is just jewelry (costume). But, Walmart has fun, cheap earrings, too. I am so sick of the one pair I have but my face is so thin I have to have something there. I had nice stars w/ a crystal (silverwire earrings but they dropped out.) Someone gave them to me w/out to extra rubber backs on them.

Drew called and said he's double a double-blind study with a new medication. (Univ. of Ash.) Half the groups gets the real thing and half the group gets a placebo. 2+/week he gets 20.00 bor going and taking it and being interviewed. Cool, huh? no one knows what the pill is. I desperately need some yummy warm sweats for being in this unit. It is the most air conditioned place I've ever been. Part of the reason I can't sleep is because I'm so cold.

My hair is falling out buddy. I __must__ get back on the hormones + get an excellent cut + possibly color this weekend. Got a lot of grey + ~~bare~~ bare area in the front. I'll get head-bands + ribbons to help. Part of it is because they (2 chicks) pulled it all out in the back, but the front has complete hair loss of all now growing in. Shit! I need help it looks awful. Estrogen + progesterone help your skin + hair + many other things. I was on it, it was great but when I went to wing C they overloaded it and didn't continue the order. Now they have me on an appetite stimulant — I'm just right for God' sakes! They said if I take it at night it would help calm me down. Well it doesn't! Extremely warm p.j's and a walk-man is what I need with some Enya + meditation tones. Or a long day outside walking in the sun is good. But it's freezing in here.

So I am going on a pass for 6 hrs. on Sunday to eat out, chop my hair off + color it + go to Wal-mart. I don't need any cosmetics at all except for <u>Firming Lotion</u> That, I have to get at a good, good store by Chanel or Lancome or Esteé Lauder. That's something you could help me with + that's all; the rest is all taken care of.

I like the glittery, translucent kind I use now. My girlfriend gave it to me for 2 shirts but it's a French brand. The CVS, + walmart don't carry something quite that specific; just moisturizers, please look around for me. K/o

I have a shower + bathroom just outside my door + loads of gels. Just no perfume. I'll get that for myself. I like Halston + they have that at Walmart - maybe even a set to wear very lightly. Shit I have the best at home - well, in storage. Paul Battobis the greatest person!. He ended up not charging me at all for the 9 mos. I paid to him while I was in here plus he had his guys put all my stuff in the shed for free storage! amezing, amazing help and compassion. I'll have to have some stuff dry cleaned and done at a big laundramat but guess what?! He owns the laundremat 1 block from my old apartment and I can hire someone to look after it for like 5.00 per large basket. I've got 6 huge plastic boxes w/ secure tops to transport the shit in when I get out. I've said he'll help me. It won't be hard. I just want my stereo, TV, + velv + victorian lamps + crystal pieces to be okay. sometimes it's fun to go through and see what you've had and forgotten. I hope mom + dad's picture + yours in those very good frames are intact.

It's so good to get away from the nasty, lazy black staff and the sloppy, vulgar, violent patients.

As for my meds which will be subject to change I take Sorbitol at night as a special laxative to reduce ammonia + detoxfy the liver. I take Metamucil morning or night. It works better at night w/ a huge bottle of warm water after. 1500 mg. of Depakote, which I need more of and Ativan 2 mg am and pm. Vistaril or Thorazine as a prn. I see the doctor today and want to ask him about increasing the Depakote + using Thorazine for sleep. It works great.

My roommate, though, is a fat, nosey black chick. She sleeps all the time + I need so I ignore her. I don't trust her for one minute. y' know talks about education — there's 6 women here + 12 guys. The guys are cool and kind of together, no problems. we smoke outside and tell jokes. I've never been involved w/ anyone here but will always remember and have a crush on Jimmy Moran. Very handsome, red-hair, tall. Went to Fordham Univ. for journalism + law. But depression + drugs got to him. He went to the Carrier Foundation from here for more ECT. Now that's a luxury hospital. I will never forget him + I will always try to find him. But somebody here told me he was dead. I had a horrible night's sleep so I've got to talk to the datoc — leave a note for the nurse that my irritability + insomnia is increasing. I need to be able to get out in the warmth and walk extensively.

So if you can — research birming lotion and preferably in a plastic bottle or they'll use it up but that's ok I have 5 things in a special box of my name on it. Time to move on out!

I love you!
Betsy
And I'll pay you back

☆ Estée Lauder Night Repair is excellent.

Release from Greystone

While Betsy was living at Greystone, I spoke to her as often as I could and, in so doing, released my parents from the stress. At one point I received a call from one of the administrators, who wanted to have a family meeting with the psychiatrists, a social worker, and other staff to discuss Betsy's future. I was shocked when the woman told me several very upsetting facts:

- Greystone was not a facility for prescription medication abusers.
- Betsy was always seeking medications and was noncompliant.
- They were not going to continue to house her indefinitely.
- They were going to remove her from all the medications she was on.

And then they shocked me by asking, "Can you pick her up or can we send her to Florida?" at which point I said, "Absolutely not," and explained why. They got the message and told me that eventually they would be discharging her.

In or around 2007, another administrator at Greystone called me and advised me that Betsy was being released. She was to be taken to Hackensack, New Jersey, where social services had found her an apartment to live in, and I was told that her Social Security Disability benefit would pay for the housing.

My husband and I flew to New Jersey, picked her up at Greystone, instead of her being transferred by taxi or a medical van, and took her to the partially furnished, barely inhabitable, one-bedroom apartment. It was a gray, gloomy, and run-down apartment building in downtown Hackensack. Betsy's demeanor and behavior was almost normal, and I surmised that this was because they had taken her off most of her medications. She appeared scared and worried, and so was I. Frank and I did not think she could make it there, living all alone, with no transportation, very little spending money, and no friends. We bought her some bedding, a winter coat, and other necessities, took her out to eat a few times, and returned to Florida. I felt more sorry for her then than at any other time in my life. I thought, "How is she going to make it all alone?" Where she would be living was one step above skid row.

In the various places she had lived prior to Greystone and to meeting and marrying Joe, she had friends to converse with, security, three meals per day, and other resources. At the efficiency apartment, she had nothing but herself. I filled our father in on the details. I was dealing with the terrible loss of my mom and his sadness about Betsy. I thought how blessed our mother was to not know about Betsy's new living situation.

A week or so later, I received a call from the psychiatric unit of a hospital in Hackensack. Betsy had been admitted there after having been caught shoplifting at the drugstore that was within walking distance of her apartment. The police were called and must have taken her directly to the hospital instead of booking her into jail. Once again, I was distraught, in tears, sick to my stomach, very angry at the system, and thought, "Now what?"

The social workers at the hospital provided me with

information about group homes and assisted living facilities, but none were affordable; most started at well over $3,000 per month. I also knew that my father was not going to subsidize her beyond the amount of money he was providing, even though my mother's Social Security benefit ended upon her death. My father and I determined that we would have to provide some assistance, but not for places in the surrounding towns in New Jersey.

Luckily, in 2008 the social worker found her a place to live in Spring Valley, New York, which was a short drive north. My husband and I flew to New Jersey, rented a car, and picked her up,

but before driving to Spring Valley, New York, we opened a bank account for her. It was not an easy process because of how the banking system requirements had changed since the terrorist attack on 9/11. The only official identification cards Betsy had were two State of New Jersey motor vehicle cards issued on November 30, 2001, which were then replaced with one issued on May 20, 2008. Upon close examination I noted two other dates (2005 and 2012) which was confusing to me

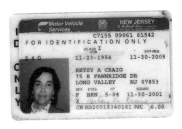

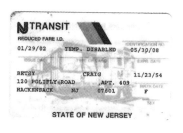

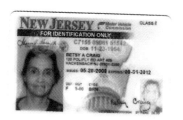

and I could tell that Betsy looked much different and older than her chronological age. The first card was issued in 2001 but expired in 2005. The reason I point this out is that when she arrived in New Jersey in 2001, she looked very attractive, and by 2008, the year she moved to Spring Valley, New York, her appearance was much different. See the following images of Betsy. The many years of her illness had taken a toll on her looks.

Despite having the three pieces of official identification, I had great difficulty opening a bank account with Bank of America for Betsy. This situation was somewhat stressful because I had become Betsy's payee for her Social Security Disability checks, and she had several that needed to be deposited. She was so lucky to have Frank and me helping her, and she was very grateful.

After her account was set up, we headed to New York and to Evergreen Court in Spring Valley. Our hope was that she would like it and be admitted, and she was. We were elated, and she seemed happy.

Evergreen Court (Spring Valley, New York) and Some Stability in Her Life

When Betsy moved into Evergreen Court, her life became more stable, at least in terms of never again being evicted and having activities to do. She also made several friends, many of whom she retained while she was living there. But sadly, a few of them moved to other facilities, and a few others died.

I was required to provide a $2,750 deposit, which was only refundable when she left the facility. At the time, Evergreen Court was not categorized as an assisted living facility.

From 2008 on, I visited her at least twice a year and always took her out to lunch and dinner. This was one of the few joys in her life, so I did not spare any expense. The picture below was taken at one of her favorite Italian restaurants in Nanuet, New York. I would also pay for takeout din-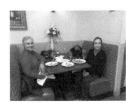ners for her long-term boyfriend, Frank, who, sadly, died about six months prior to the March 23, 2021, fire, which I will discuss later in some detail.

Sundays with Dunkin' Donuts and Shopping

As mentally draining, painful, and taxing as it often was to travel from Florida to New Jersey, I always looked forward to seeing Betsy and her friends, particularly on Sundays with the Dunkin' Donuts items I bought. Every time I visited her, I went to the local Dunkin' Donuts and bought three to four dozen doughnuts, coffee, creamer, sugar, and other condiments for the residents. They looked forward to my visits, and I enjoyed sitting outside and chatting with them. Sometimes I would join Betsy for lunch in the main dining room and go to the different tables to say hello, always reminding myself that they were human beings who once had normal lives. *There but by the grace of God go I.*

My visits to Betsy gave some joy to many residents who had no family or whose families had abandoned them or rarely visited them. I believe that speaking with them made a difference in their lives. Betsy would sometimes tell me before a visit that several residents had asked about me and were looking forward to my visit.

I also looked forward to taking Betsy for pedicures and manicures, giving her spending money, and buying her clothes, often secondhand from Goodwill and sometimes new. She loved shopping at the Goodwill store in Nanuet, and I enjoyed helping her pick out items she liked. I also paid extra so she could have a private room before the facility became an ACLF, at which time it became more affordable. For many years, Frank and I paid over $1,100 for the private room.

Below is a picture of some of the residents, which they allowed me to take after we all enjoyed doughnuts and coffee.

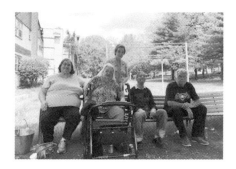

06

Overview

After reading the book *Hidden Victims Hidden Healers: An Eight-Stage Healing Process for Families and Friends of the Mentally Ill*, authored by Julie Tallard Johnson, I decided to add the "four Cs." Thank you, Julie, for your remarkable insight and ability to put this information into words and for providing me with additional motivation to write this book.

How you and your family have been able to deal with the terrible situations your mentally ill loved one gets into should give you insight into how well you can accept the following:

- You cannot cure it.
- You didn't cause it.
- You cannot control it.
- You must cope with it.

The four Cs greatly helped me and enabled our parents and me to continue with our lives, assist Betsy, and accept that tomorrow was another day. We did what alcoholics are taught to do: live one day at a time. The struggle for us was not living our lives and always having Betsy in the front of our minds—the tragedy of her and for her.

I believe that if you read about the four Cs, you will be in a better position to deal with and solve some of your own emotional struggles. Repeating the four Cs to yourself will help you when dealing with the most recent major, debilitating event. Having faith in and relying on the four Cs will greatly benefit you. Compare each C to a Band-Aid, which helps to heal the pain, wherein each C can be your defense mechanism against the pain your loved one suffers and transfers onto you.

You Did Not Cause It

Remember, "You didn't cause it." The illness is genetic. Based on research and case studies of families, there is an identified genetic link. Even though my parents knew that my father's grandmother was eccentric, they didn't have the faintest clue that one of their children could be born with bipolar disorder.

Regarding the decision of whether to have children, there are also false positives and false negatives. Let me use an example of a prison inmate to explain this. The inmate completes his psychological tests (e.g., the Minnesota Multiphasic Personality Inventory or the California Psychological Inventory), and the forensic psychologist analyzes the results and the written report. Based on the psychologist's analysis, the test results predict that the inmate is unlikely to kill again and should be released. However, once released, the inmate harms his grandparents.

You could be told by a genetics expert that there is a 40 to 60 percent chance (this is my estimate) that if you have a child, he or she may carry the gene for bipolar disorder. The tests could produce false positives or false negatives. I don't think any married couple would be happy about bringing a child into the world who might become mentally ill. Although the couple has the right to decide what is best for them, they might be better off adopting a child. So the bottom line here is that *you did not cause it!*

However, there are other factors involved. As covered earlier, there are the genetic, environmental, and psychological/emotional links. In terms of the psychological/emotional link, for example, you may have caused some anguish for your loved one by not being compassionate or understanding enough or may not have handled a tragedy as well as you could have. Nevertheless, the longer you deal with the person's mental illness, the more important it is that you continue to remind yourself that you did not cause the illness.

Some contextual factors, such as friends of your loved one using drugs and drinking alcohol, more than likely exacerbated your loved one's illness. It is best to be an attentive observer. The way you treat your loved one can trigger a negative episode, more so than with a person who is not afflicted with genetic-based mood swings. Therefore, you need to be on guard and be ready at any time to tread lightly when the individual appears to be in a manic or depressed state of mind.

There are other factors that may intervene and can cause a manic or depressed episode for the individual. Constant change in location and type of housing, lack of safety and security, need for medications that the person does not have, or not having enough health insurance can cause a manic or depressed episode.

You Cannot Control It

Remember, "You cannot control it." That's right; you definitely cannot control the illness nor the person's stability or instability on their drugs. You cannot control their mood swings. You cannot control: the poor decisions they make, despite offering your opinion; how they behave in the hospital; how they are treated in the hospital; or what treatment they receive or do not receive. You may have a voice, but you cannot control it.

Caregivers should be aware that that many mentally ill people do not take their medications when they are feeling good and subsequently become unstable again. You can ask yourself over and over, "Why won't they stay on the medicine?" or "Why does he or she under- or overmedicate?" But asking such questions will not solve the problem. One strategy I often used was to put myself in my sister's shoes and imagine how it felt to experience so many side effects from the medications: nausea, headaches, loss of appetite, weight gain, weight loss, dry mouth, dizziness, lethargy, blurred vision, and constipation. I did my best to understand why she was the type of person doctors would label as "medication seeking." I attributed this behavior to her impulsivity, her addictive personality, and her belief that she knew better than some of the doctors. For example, she would say: "No, I am not seeking painkillers; I am in bad pain."

You also cannot control how a person's system will react to new medications, a new doctor, a change in medication routine, or a stay at a hospital, hundreds of miles away, which will put stress on you because of the travel time and cost. You will have little control over how they manage their lives and how much they will require your assistance, which may include dealing with legal issues. In my sister's case, one time, as I said, I had to plead with a store's security officer to not arrest my sister for stealing. I was unaware that she had stuffed some clothes inside her jacket. You also will not be able to control whether your loved one will get arrested, particularly if you are not there when they are caught and are in the process of being arrested.

Overall, you cannot control their chemical imbalance or how their brain is reacting to a specific medication. You certainly can't control whether they decide to allow their current psychiatrist or medical doctor to provide you with any information, and when you get information from them, whether it is the truth. Under the Health Insurance Portability and Accountability Act of 1996 (HIPPA), a patient has the right to tell a doctor to not give you any information.

You also cannot control the mental health system, the level or quality of services provided in each state, or whether your loved one will receive services at all.

A letter Betsy wrote to me about one of the inpatient psychiatric hospitals reflects the lack of control I had over this aspect of her life.

Dear Linse, (my meds were doubled!)
Now my two numbers
at this fucking dump
are 822-3754 or
✗ ✗ 822-3754 are code
(813). I share the room
with a bitchy woman
with pulmonary disease
and parakeets - I got like
4 hours sleep. They
sing all night. I
really got screwed here -
they moved me w/out mom's
permission - roaches + disabled. at least I can walk
alot. My head is so disorgan-

ized I can barely see a way out. Daddy keeps yelling that the system will take care of me. Listen, please try to send me a cashier's check. No one will cash checks for me except maybe Publix and it's like 8 mi. away. I had to pay 179.— out of Drew's $ for meds 'cuz, they couldn't wait 2 days for a photocopy from HAS

I NEED
A WATCH

BADLY

CUTE
CHEAP
SPARKLY

Look just call 'cuz now is group, walk to post office, sleep, Call. Please, esp after 6. love me.

Please note that you *can* control how you react to your loved one's illness and difficulties, which is half the battle. As you continue to live with the illness, you will soon grow accustomed to what you can and cannot control.

When I assumed full-time caregiving services for my sister, I got used to her regular crisis phone calls and calls requesting money, and when she was having a good day, sometimes she would even ask me how I was doing. There were a few years of security and stability, when she was living at Evergreen Court in Spring Valley, New York. This provided me with a sense of relief and serenity; I knew that she would not end up on the streets, because the State of New York does not allow assisted living facilities to evict a resident without finding the person another suitable place to live.

Many doctors advised Betsy and me that she was a rapid cycler. In other words, her mood swings were sometimes every twenty-four hours, weekly, and/or monthly. I prayed, on many occasions, that new medications would slow down her mood swings, but unfortunately, this rarely happened.

Please do not delude yourself into thinking that mental illness is reserved for the poor, people of color, common criminals, newly arrived legal or undocumented immigrants, or people who live on the streets of America. Mental illnesses affect people from all races and social classes. If you search the internet, you will discover many famous people and celebrities who have been diagnosed as having a mental disorder. The list includes celebrities such as Mariah Carey, Robert Downey Jr., Ted Turner, Mel Gibson, and Catherine Zeta-Jones. You must accept the fact that you cannot control your loved one's illness. I finally accepted the cold, hard reality that I would never, ever be able to control Betsy's illness. It was a long trip of denial.

You Cannot Cure It

Providing financial and emotional support, companionship, and a permanent place to live, Evergreen Court, from 2008 to 2022, did not cure her illness. But medications did help her, if and when she took them as prescribed.

Although the scientific community has been able to send men to the moon, cure some childhood leukemias, create children through in vitro fertilization, clone sheep, build the internet, design and deploy artificial intelligence applications, and invent new products, the brilliant minds of the world have not been able to, and probably may never totally be able to, fully cure diseases of the brain. Based on my lay knowledge and having seen pictures, the brains of the mentally ill are structured differently. My sister was brilliant but seriously mentally ill.

You must remember that you cannot cure or mediate the illness—you can only be supportive and available to your loved one. You can, however, hope and pray for the day the medical profession finds other medications that will provide a longer stabilization for people such as my sister and your loved one. You can work toward and pray for the day when the politicians in Washington and the insurance companies finally start treating mental illnesses as they do other medical conditions and provide the appropriate funding levels for research and treatment. I am being pessimistic, but I strongly feel that even though the

United States is facing an even greater health care crisis after the pandemic, funding levels will not be increased.

The burden to taxpayers is exorbitant. If more mentally ill people had the funding for treatment with medication and affordable health insurance, they might be able to become productive members of society. It is better to be productive than to be a burden to families and to the taxpayers, who also must be financially responsible and resent doing so. State and federal funds are often wasted on needless programs and pork-barrel congressional projects and not spent on the mental health of citizens.

You Must Cope with It

The last C is, for you, one of the most important of the Cs, due to its relevance to your mental and physical well-being. Remember that totally cutting your loved one off from any contact is a drastic way of coping. My sincere belief is that most families who come to the realization that they are dealing with someone who has a brain disease will attempt to cope with the illness instead of abandoning the person. I hope you understand that our family's trauma was self-imposed, due to our love of Betsy. Each family must identify its own short- and long-term coping goals.

As I previously mentioned, one of the strategies for coping is similar to what alcoholics who attend AA meetings have to do: live one day at a time. Essentially, that's what you must do. Instead of planning for your loved one's future, unless it is related to how they will be provided for once you have passed on or to estate planning, you should just cope with their illness and crises on a day-to-day basis. Consider your goals and remember that there is always tomorrow. After you have gone through many tragic experiences with a mentally ill person, you must adjust and deal with the reality of their life. The latter comment may seem trite; however, the reality is that the more situations you have had to deal with, the better you will be able to cope with the next one. One step at a time. One day at a time.

During all my visits to see Betsy, I coped by spending hours alone thinking and reflecting about our visit, her life, and where I could take her so we could have some enjoyment. During one of my visits, she was living at Evergreen Court, Spring Valley, New York, and was sent to the Northern Riverview Hospital and Rehabilitation facility in Haverstraw, New York, which is about a thirty-minute drive from Spring Valley. Unfortunately, I canceled my reservation at the Hampton Inn in Nanuet, New York, and chose a bed-and-breakfast that was within walking distance from the Northern Riverview Hospital in Haverstraw, New York.

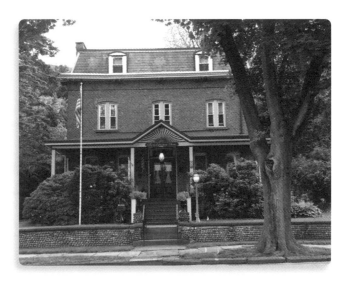

I always wanted to be as close to her as possible and to not have to call so many Lyft drivers. I stopped renting cars because the process was adding too much stress to my already busy weekend visits.

I searched and found a nice resort restaurant, the Water Club, on the Hudson River and an Italian restaurant on Route 9. I visited the Water Club or more than one occasion, including the year she passed on, and the Italian restaurant during the last year of Betsy's life. Both visits helped me relax and made me happy. However, both times Betsy was unable to go with me, as she was not 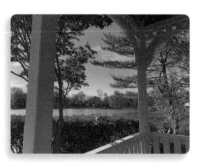 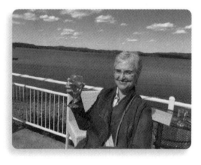 allowed to leave the Northern River Hospital.

On one visit, when I decided to walk to the Water Club, I left the bed-and-breakfast, walked down the hill, and enjoyed watching the ducks.

I always took time to engage in activities that made me happy, because if I only stayed in the hotels in Nanuet and Nyack, or the bed-and-breakfast in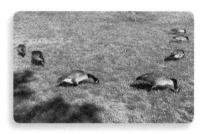

Haverstraw, I would be sad.

On one visit we took a cab with Betsy's boyfriend, Frank, to visit her friend Barbara, who had moved to Pine Valley, a very nice assisted living facility in Spring Valley, New York. We ordered pizza. Barbara was a nurse for her entire adult life; was, at one time, married; and had a few children. However, she got divorced, was diagnosed with bipolar disorder, and ended up living in ACLFs. I do not know whether she got divorced because of the illness. I never asked her, because I did not want to intrude on her personal life.

In summary, think about an armadillo, which has a leathery armor shell that protects it from predators when it rolls up into a ball. You will eventually grow your outer shell, 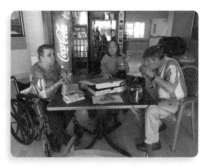 which will help you to cope! You must be the person who asks and answers the question: How willing are you to commit to continue to surround your mentally ill family member with love? The choice is yours, and only you can choose how you will act or react.

THE STAGES OF HEALING AND SOME COPING STRATEGIES

07

Overview

The stages described in this chapter are not found in any medical textbook, published articles, or other literature. The stages are based on my years of dealing with my sister's illness. I carefully thought about what my parents and I experienced, and I named and documented the phases accordingly.

Disbelief and Denial

When my sister was first diagnosed with a mental disorder, I was in a complete state of denial, but it was true. Back in 1975, her disorder was referred to as manic depression. My total ignorance of the illness, my youth, and my inexperience contributed to this thought process: "How could this be true? No, not my sister, the beautiful, athletic, funny, and brilliant woman who is attending an Ivy League university!"

We don't really comprehend what occurs in the mind of a mentally ill person. We can only imagine, and psychiatrists and/or pharmacologists can only treat the symptoms. There were many ways in which my sister dealt with her illness. She continuously used denial or projection techniques. After years of dealing with this behavior, I was finally able to understand why she denied that she was ill and/or blamed me or someone else.

She was in the denial phase for several years. Eventually, my parents and I finally realized that we were dealing with an incurable and lifelong illness. As the years progressed, and when she was still able to work and finish college and graduate school, my thoughts included: She'll be OK once she finds the right medication; This can't be . . . she used to be so vibrant; No, not my sister, not my family . . . this too shall pass; and Once she finds the right man and a job that is not stressful, she'll be all right. These types of thoughts continued over the years. They were all rationalizations; I was trying to block the real truth.

Our parents never told any of their friends or neighbors and hid their daughter's illness in the closet. They did not want anyone to know why an adult woman was living at home. However, when they moved to their new home in Florida in 1987 and made new friends (during which time Betsy was still living with them), they opened the door and told close friends the truth. I remember my mother saying, "We aren't hiding this anymore. I am not lying to people anymore about what's wrong with my daughter. It's out in the open now. I am not going to make up stories as to why she doesn't work."

My father never denied or disbelieved she was ill. He just didn't understand the manifestations of this type of mental disorder, he did not like to discuss it, and he did not demonstrate much sympathy. He denied that most of her behavior was due to the illness and instead blamed her behavior on past drug use.

Based on my knowledge gleaned from many books and articles about mental illness, many people with a mental disorder use drugs to sedate their mood swings. Because our father was very pragmatic and task oriented, he took the actions necessary to effectively deal with each situation. But he used to believe that Betsy's impulsivity was what caused her to get into trouble, get evicted from apartments, get arrested for shoplifting, lose friends, etcetera. He finally realized that lack of self-control was part of her illness.

In summary, moving from the disbelief and denial phase eventually occurs, and it helped my parents and me. However, considering society's general ignorance about and lack of acceptance of mental illness, even so many years after my sister's diagnosis in 1975, I recommend that you be careful whom you tell about your loved one's illness, because it could affect your friendships. Another drastic thing that could happen is that if there is a break-in in your neighborhood, one or more of your neighbors may tell the police, "The mentally ill person who lives at X address probably did it." Therefore, protecting your privacy might be the best decision you could make. It is really contingent upon where you are living and your interactions and history with your neighbors. You must analyze the situation before taking action. One step at a time.

Anxiety

Anyone who has been depressed knows that it cannot be readily identified if the person represses feelings and does not demonstrate abnormal behavior. Only recently have I had the insight to know that my problem with low self-esteem was mostly caused by growing up with, and living as an adult with, a mentally ill sister. Her verbal abuse and manipulation continued until her death. What frightened me the most, over the years, was worrying that Betsy's depressed moods could result in a successful suicide.

As a caregiver and support system for my parents, I knew that I could never afford to get sick. The caregiver cannot afford to get sick because they will be of no use to themself or their loved one. Unfortunately, our mother got to the point that her worry and anxiety evolved into depression. But somehow, she developed the ability to snap herself out of depression.

Overall, please don't allow your worry and anxiety to devour you. The key is accepting and understanding that you will have these feelings frequently, and that at times, it will negatively impact your life. It should be only a temporary situation. It is something you should understand. You also need to keep in mind that you are the caregiver to your loved one, and constant worry and anxiety can affect your own mental well-being.

Guilt

We all know that guilt is an unhealthy emotion to hold on to. However, not ever feeling guilt is unrealistic and generally attributed to those with sociopathic behavior. Guilt is one of the phases I have gone through, particularly early in my sister's illness. I felt guiltier when my sister moved to New Jersey and then New York in 2008 because I could not be there in person to help her. However, had she been living near me, my life might have been totally disrupted and unmanageable.

One example of the guilt I felt about Betsy's illness was that she never went on any nice vacations. Therefore, I never told her about any of the vacations I took with my husband, Frank—including a millennium cruise, other cruises, a three-week trip to France in 1992, and numerous trips to Key West. I felt that it was cruel and that she may have perceived that I was intentionally making her feel bad. Whenever she asked me what Frank and I were doing or going to do, I would focus on our exercising and spending time with friends or his daughters.

I also felt very guilty and extremely sad over her estrangement from our parents and that after she moved to New Jersey in 2001, she never saw them again. Sometimes I ruminated about this but did my best to calm my mind and move on to other thoughts.

As I continued to learn more about the illness, through reading books and articles, attending NAMI meetings, remembering the experiences I had with a former bipolar friend, conversing with our parents about their dealings with my sister, and, of course, attending my own therapy sessions, I was able to let go of the guilt over my sister having the illness instead of me.

Frankly, I became tired of beating myself up over something that I finally realized I could not control. Once I learned about the three Cs and added my own fourth C—"You must cope with it"—I was finally able to work on freeing myself of the guilt over why it was her and not me. Our mother also had great difficulty with guilty feelings. Over the years, she had asked herself many questions, such as: Was I not a good enough mother? Was I too lenient with my husband and the way he detached from my daughter's situation? Did all the moves contribute to her illness? Should they have put her on a medication treatment when she was using drugs and before she overdosed in 1975? I believe that my mother just didn't know what was wrong with Betsy until her daughter had her first drug overdose, which resulted in a three-month stay in Butler Hospital at Brown University.

Questions will go round and round in your mind, and you will probably ask yourself a great many of the same types of questions. Don't let this concern you. You must just accept that you will initially feel a great deal of guilt, but try to train your mind to not allow you to beat yourself up with guilt.

Since 1975, I thought about my sister every day and always remembered what a dreadful and sad life she led and felt deeply sorry for her. My feelings of guilt mostly emerged when I thought about how grateful I was about how my life turned out.

Guilt is not only an unhealthy feeling that causes you anxiety and pain, but it is also often a useless feeling. It washes away whatever psychic energy you have. I know. I used to feel guilt-ridden, and I spent much effort repressing the thoughts so as not to diminish my psychic energy and intellectual abilities. Freeing myself of guilt did not occur overnight; it took many years of soul searching and reflection. Some residual guilt will remain with me for the rest of my life.

Overall, while you deal with your loved one's illness, you will experience feelings of guilt more often than you would imagine. It is natural to feel guilty, but don't let it take over your life to such an extent that you cause yourself a degree of stress that has a negative impact on you mentally and physically. As I said previously, if you are sick, you will not be able to provide the caregiving service to your loved one, much less yourself and your other family members.

Anger

I am still angry about the lack of public support and recognition that results in mental illness costing society millions of dollars. I am deeply concerned about the way mentally ill patients are treated by the system. I am angry at the fact that they are only treated for as long as the number of hospital days in their bank, and once the days are used up or expire, they are kicked out. Being angry about the lack of facilities and lack of regular and consistent medical help for your loved one is a natural feeling. If you haven't ever been angry, you have not experienced, in totality, the effects of dealing and living with a mentally ill person. Don't despair; anger is just another feeling that provides you with the impetus to continue to "hang in there," and provide continued support to your loved one. Anger is also to be expected on a fairly continuous basis, particularly after having to deal with the afflicted person's verbal abuse and escapades. You must be able to allow compassion to smother your anger.

My parents and I were angry about my sister's lack of concern or understanding about how her behavior negatively impacted other people. We were angry over how the system works and, for that matter, how it doesn't work, and how, after she used up her hospital days, she'd be released with little or no follow-up until the next major incident. We were angry over the lack of decent housing for her and for other mentally ill people. We were angry when people who lived in the same complex she was living in called the property manager to try to get rid of her or called the police about her bizarre behavior. One place where she lived even had an attorney representing the management write an abusive and critical letter to our parents, threatening them with eviction and legal action if my sister's behavior was not controlled. However, considering the circumstances, I could not blame them, but I was still terribly angry. You must recognize your anger and not let it consume the good in you, because your primary responsibility is to help your loved one.

Anger cuts both ways; it is directed toward the ill person and toward the system. It can also be directed toward other family members who may not be coping well on a particular day. Anger is a continual phase that may dissipate shortly after an incident, depending upon how serious and mentally debilitating it was.

Accept the fact that on many occasions you will feel anger; it is a natural feeling that should not cause you guilt. Just make whatever effort you can to direct the anger at something other than yourself.

Fear

For years I feared the death of my sister through suicide and what might become of her in an unprotected environment. My mother was also worried about this; there were times when we would cry together. I feared that Betsy would one day be incarcerated in one of the terrible state psychiatric hospitals. Unfortunately, the old "insane asylum" may still exist in some form in a number of states. She was placed in a terrible one when she lived at Greystone Psychiatric Hospital in Morris Plains, New Jersey, for two years. However, based on what I learned about it, the environment could have been much worse.

As noted previously, I feared that she could end up on the streets, but fortunately this never happened. As I said, it did not occur because our parents and I were there to be her caregivers.

While I was finishing and editing this manuscript, I wanted to find out the number of mentally ill people who are living on the streets or in our jails and prisons. Some of the statistics were astounding.

In summary, fear is one of the most debilitating phases you will undoubtedly pass through. It can, however, drive you to do more positive and productive things with your life and when you are helping your mentally ill loved one. Channel your fear. Do not let it consume you. Wake up each morning to a new day. One day at a time.

Misunderstanding

It wasn't until I attended NAMI meetings and read literature discussing bipolar disorder and other mental disorders that I was able to better understand how horrible and debilitating the illness is. Some of the stories other family members told at the meetings were horrific and heart wrenching, but as the years rolled on, my understanding came to comfort me.

Misunderstanding comes in the form of forgetting that the lashing-out behavior is part of the illness and should not be cause for you to get sick, angry, or upset. However, often times

I was not in control of my emotions. Misunderstanding also occurs when you are critical of the person and say to yourself, as I did on many occasions, "I don't understand why she is being this way," or "Why did she do that? Doesn't she know it's wrong and irrational?"

As I experienced more of my sister's horrible episodes, I compartmentalized them into my memory bank. I found out that no matter how angry or upset I got about whatever incident Betsy had just experienced (having an accident in the main bathroom at Evergreen Court the day she was moving there, being called by the state highway patrol to tell me that my sister was found standing on the side of the road, pleading with the general manager at Evergreen Court to allow Besty to stay there even though she had been caught smoking in her room on two occasions), a few hours later, she remembered very little, if any, of what had occurred. I used to think she was lying or deliberately got herself into trouble when she told me she did not remember the incident. However, she did remember the times she got caught smoking but lied about it anyway. But I finally learned that, due to the illness, she really did not recall what caused most incidents. I also grew to understand that when Betsy's medications were not working was when some of the episodes occurred.

Another part of misunderstanding is saying to yourself, "Why did she or he have to say that? Why did she or he shoplift? Why is she or he lying?" Asking these questions is not productive behavior on your part. The sooner you accept that "What is, is," the better off you will be. I also told myself on many occasions,

"I don't know why she's treating me and my parents this way, and why isn't she more grateful for what we do for her" and then I finally shifted to trying to understand what she was going through.

We had no idea that the illness would grow worse as the years wore on, but we ultimately understood that part of the problem was that we kept rescuing her. However, because of the limited resources in Florida for the mentally ill, we had no other choice but to continue to help Betsy as much as we could. Fortunately, we learned to put our negative emotions aside, stop crying, and deal with the crises in a pragmatic manner. We also learned that money did not solve the problem. For example, a nicer apartment, which my parents subsidized, made no difference at all.

In summary, becoming more educated about mental illness will provide you with a better understanding. Additionally, continually learning that scientists are constantly formulating and testing new medications that may help and reading all you can about mental illness should give you some hope for tomorrow, the tomorrow when your loved one may be able to live a better life. We all should try to live with hope.

A depressive illness is not just a "case of the blues" but a severe and persistent biological disease. The two most common types of depressive illness are unipolar (characterized by deep, prolonged depression) and bipolar or manic depression (characterized by cycles of deep depression and inappropriate highs).[16]

---

16. NAMI brochure, 1993.

Acceptance

The phase of acceptance will come slowly and after many years of dealing with your mentally ill loved one. For some of you, it may be too difficult to grasp, which is perfectly understandable. But we must hope that we will eventually be able to accept what is. For those of you who have reached this point or are slowly reaching it, you will probably attain a sense of peace and happiness. This is because you will have spent much time reading and will finally realize that mental illness is a reality, that it does truly exist, and that your loved one is, in fact, diagnosed with a mental illness. Why do I say that you will attain a sense of peace and happiness? Because until you reach the point of acceptance, you will never be able to move on to the phase of healing. Once you finally accept that the person is mentally ill and not in control of his or her behavior, you will be better equipped to deal with their illness and how you react to them.

Of course, accepting their various aberrations and negative behaviors, particularly their verbal abuse, is not easy and causes much stress. However, you need to accept the illness that they inherited or that may have been partially manifested by some major tragedy in their lives or by prolonged drug abuse. You need to accept that their mental illness is the reality of their life. It is the reality that you, as a parent, will have to face or you, as a sibling or spouse, will no doubt have to deal with from time to time. Accepting your loved one for what they are is difficult and often not a pleasant situation. Again, it is absolutely essential for you to accept that you cannot cure it or control it and that you did not cause it.

Acceptance is also related to how society and the public health care system work to help both you and your loved one with the illness. Getting angry is OK and natural, but refusing to accept the cold, cruel reality of an insufficient public health care system for the mentally ill and others in need, whose family insurance policies will no longer cover catastrophic illnesses such as mental illness, will not help you at all. You must learn to accept the system for all its failings and use your cognitive abilities, patience, and understanding to work with it and learn as much as you can about what is out there to assist you and the mentally ill person.

Accepting your loved one as a person is also particularly important, because she or he is a living human being. Accepting them as they are will also provide you and them with a chance to enjoy some quality time together and to make some positive, if truly short term, goals for their future.

Hope

Hope is one of the phases that is continually intermingled with all of the other phases. It is the one phase that enabled me and my parents to go on to the next day. I always held the belief that if we do not have hope, we do not have anything. I hoped for new miracle medications that would further stabilize bipolar patients and be affordable to most patients. I hoped for additional funding for research and for group homes for the mentally ill, and I hoped that my sister would eventually find some semblance of peace in her life. I hoped that someday she would finally recognize and decide to deal with her addiction to some of the medications and drugs, then do something about it. That day came way too late in her life. I also hoped that she would experience some happiness and joy in her life. When you are a caregiver, hope should be the bedrock of your behavior.

In summary, please remember that hope is what will keep you going and provide you with the impetus to remain strong and capable of coping with the ongoing tragedies. Hope allows you to believe that maybe tomorrow or the next year, or the year after, there will be better days for the lives of the mentally ill in this society, who could, if they were in control of their behavior, be productive and happy members of society. Also, you must understand that we live at a time when the mentally ill are rejected by many facets of society. We are also living at a time when mental-illness issues are much more out of the closet than they were fifty years ago, due to the internet and social media.

It's obvious that mental health centers prefer to treat patients who are passive, compliant, and have Medicaid! How can persons with mental illness who are listed as a priority clients be denied services because they don't fit some staff member's profile?[17]

---

17. NAMI Sun, 1993.

MORE COPING STRATEGIES 08

Overview

When I recall the many years of my sister's illness, I realize that my parents and I each had our own way of coping. This section of the book is about the ways I learned to cope; some became strategies because of the sometimes ineffective way I was coping. One example of my ineffective coping was that I would raise my voice at my sister, which often would end up with both of us hanging up the phone. I hope the strategies that follow help you.

Do Not Sacrifice Your Own Needs

Coping with the illness and its effects on family members is critical. If you do not keep yourself healthy and rested, you will be of little use to the ill family member. My advice to you is not to sacrifice your own needs at the expense of your mentally ill family member. If you are not of a sound, stable mind and health, you will not be able to be a caregiver to your family member. Yes, their needs, at times, are greater than yours but addressing them should not be at the expense of your needs and mental health. Your needs must be satisfied before you can deal with the situation. Anger does not help, nor does lashing back. I've learned this the hard way when anger seemed to repress my love for Betsy. Remember, we are not only continually coping with our family member's illness and providing for their needs, but we are also dealing with our own lives, families, children, work, friends, and extracurricular activities.

Do Not Lose Your Temper

Raising your voice, sometimes yelling, hanging up the phone, or lashing out at your loved one does not help the situation. Stay in control, and do not lose your temper. I lost my temper too many times to remember and always regretted it afterward.

I remember so many times when Betsy would be so pushy and aggressive to me while we were having a phone conversation that I would raise my voice. The conversation would end with one of us hanging up the phone. Oftentimes my husband would hear the conversation and tell me to stop raising my voice and would remind me that I would only be upset afterward. He was always correct.

Do Not Fall Apart

Our mother was a very strong, patient, caring, and resilient person, and because of her, the family unit never completely fell apart. Crying was one of the emotions that prevented my mother and me from falling apart. Falling apart could be having a nervous breakdown, having a car accident, or getting drunk and being arrested for a DUI. Fortunately, this never happened to me or my mother. My mother was like the Rock of Gibraltar. But being the Rock of Gibraltar took its toll on her. I am surprised she was able to cope as long as she did before she was diagnosed with congestive heart failure in 2000 and died six years later.

Be a Caregiver, Not a Caretaker

As a parent to a mentally ill person, you must be a caregiver and not a caretaker or enabler. If your mentally ill loved one can hold down a job, encourage him or her to do so, and don't readily give him or her money. They will come to expect it. Provide your loved one with extra food, old furniture, car insurance, or used clothes. In other words, give tangible items so that they won't have cash to spend foolishly. My sister spent her money frivolously, and if she had more of it, she'd go on shopping trips and spend the money on other people. Don't allow yourself to continuously give your loved one money or underwrite their manic episodes. Put a limit on all credit cards. Use your finances for things they need that will enable them to live on their own. Financial issues, if not dealt with on a pragmatic level, can cause additional stress on the family. Having everyone provide some of the financial support—if this is a viable option for your family—takes the full burden off one person. If your loved one has a checking account or credit card, you should use a local bank. Make contact with the bank manager in order to have a live person who can monitor the account and maintain contact with this person.

Allow Time to Cry

When our mother shared her feelings with me while embracing me, we both sat and cried. She also told me that she prayed that my sister would not outlive her, as she was quite worried that Betsy might end up homeless. My mother also had difficulty sleeping some nights, because she had dreams about my sister roaming the streets once her mother was gone. This is a difficult and sad thing to discuss with your mother or any family member, but believe me, it will help you reach a more realistic acceptance level. It's better to discuss these thoughts than to let them tear you up inside.

Provide Some Financial Assistance

Looking at the bright side for a moment, I see that my sister was fortunate we were able to continually assist her financially. The amount the state provides a disabled person is below the poverty level, and this includes food stamps. I'm not saying that the state should allow these individuals to live like kings and queens, but they need to provide more financial assistance if they can't provide decent living facilities. If you are able to provide some financial assistance, you may prevent them from having to live on the streets.

When I was editing the final draft of this manuscript, I did some research on this topic. What I found is alarming:

- Half of unsheltered individuals live in California, a third of whom are estimated to have serious mental illness.[18]
- "The number of unhoused people with severe

18. Dembosky, Templeton, and Feibel, "When Homelessness and Mental Illness Overlap."

mental illness is often inflated, but nevertheless tragically high: at least 25 percent of those forced to live on the street have a diagnosis of a severe mental illness, and many more likely qualify even if they're undiagnosed."[19]

• "Of the 14 million or so people who experience the most debilitating mental health conditions, roughly one third don't receive treatment. The reasons are manifold—some forgo that treatment by choice—but far too many simply cannot connect with the services they want and need."[20]

Florida, my home state, ranks at the bottom for providing health and rehabilitative services, yet it has one of the largest bureaucracies in the United States, with over thirty-three thousand employees. I was glad that Betsy moved to New Jersey and then New York.

You must have an awareness of the programs for the mentally ill in the state where your loved one is living. Become familiar with the state agencies and do your best to prevent your loved one from becoming a statistic.

---

19. Zeb Larson, "Don't Bring Back Mental Asylums. Instead, Build the Welfare State," *Jacobin*, March 8, 2023, https://jacobin.com/2023/03/mental-asylums-welfare-state-involuntary-incarceration-hospitalization.

20. *The New York Times* Editorial Board. "The Solution to America's Mental Health Crisis Already Exists," *The New York Times*, October 4, 2022, https://www.nytimes.com/2022/10/04/opinion/us-mental-health-community-centers.html

Do Not Let the Illness Tear Your Family Unit Apart

Mental illness also has the potential to tear a family apart. It almost tore my family apart, including my marriage and my parents' fifty-six-year marriage. The potential to tear a family up doesn't occur when the person is somewhat stable and not in crisis. It's the crisis times that are extremely difficult. You never know when the last shoe will drop, so to speak, so come to grips with the illness, and try not to feel so alone.

Our parents were, for a time, enablers but then grew to become caregivers. This was the best route for them to take. If so, do it rapidly, and learn from the experience. Be in contact with relatives who live near the current abode of your loved one, in case their help is required.

Do Not Terminate Contact

At times, my parents considered terminating all contact with Betsy, because their sorrow, misunderstanding, and stress levels were too great. I told my father, "I know you never expected your retirement years to end like this. You never imagined you'd be burdened with a daughter who once had everything going for her." I also conveyed to him on many occasions that I understood the pain he felt, particularly when Betsy was out of control, lashed out at him, and called him terrible names. We promised one another we would not abandon Betsy, even though she would often blame us for our dysfunctional family and her illness. We came to understand that her behavior was due to her mental illness and not to her true, rational feelings.

It's also so easy for a parent or close sibling to want to write the person off, tune them out, detach totally, or cut them off completely. Some people may consider this to be safer, but this is not the way to deal with the situation, especially when you feel anger. As a caregiver, you must live one day at a time when it comes to dealing with your loved one, just as they are forced to live only for the day. Remember, their future is bleak. They probably will never have the same freedoms we do, experience the same happiness we do, or have a normal and secure relationship with an intimate partner. Everyone needs a lifeline, and we were Betsy's.

Try Hard to Accept Them as They Are

As a caregiver, it may take all your mental strength, perseverance, and patience to accept your loved one as she or he is. Remember, a mentally ill person does not think or feel the same way we do and therefore requires, by default, more attention and patience. They should not be expected to accept us the way we are, but we need to learn to accept them for who they are. Imagine what they have to deal with—accepting themselves for what they have become and living with this for the rest of their lives! It's a great burden, which most of us could not imagine having to deal with on a daily basis. Do not let guilt consume you. One day at a time.

Feelings of guilt, if not stopped, can cause you to become sick to your stomach, and then unhealthy bacteria may start to grow if you do not expel the feelings. If the bacteria continue to grow, they may eventually eat you from the inside out. In retrospect, if this occurs, people often begin to dislike themselves.

THE FIRE AND BEGINNING OF THE END 09

Overview

Betsy was one of the survivors of a horrifying fire that occurred at Evergreen Court, Spring Valley, New York, on March 23, 2021, and this tragic story is portrayed in this chapter. Starting on that date, her life was in a downward spiral, and I lived much of what she went through for the next eighteen months. Because many sorrowful events took place, the subsections are listed.

The Morning of March 24, 2021

I was riding my stationary recumbent bike and feeling pretty good. Pedaling, drinking coffee, and staring straight ahead is a quiet, peaceful, and meditative way for me to start the day. I checked my cell phone, and I saw that a message came in from Nancy (her last name is omitted for privacy) from Evergreen Court, in Spring Valley, New York, which was the ACLF where my sister had been living for well over fourteen years. I was told that the facility used to be a hotel—travelers would stay there on their way to upstate New York—and that it was well over one hundred years old.

Nancy's short, terse, and upsetting message was, "Hi, Linsey. There was a fire last night at Evergreen Court. Your sister is safe, but everybody has been moved to the Belvedere in downtown Brooklyn." *Click!*

I played the message back, because I couldn't believe what I had just heard. The message lacked empathy and concern and was robotic.

I called Nancy back; she answered the phone and was very harried and in a rush. I asked her to tell me about the fire. Her unbelievable and unsettling response was, "I don't know much about it, but you can look it up on the internet. All I know is your sister is OK and is in downtown Brooklyn." Given the tone of her voice, I surmised that what happened was far worse than she was revealing.

Background on Evergreen Court

Nancy was an administrator at Evergreen Court in charge of admitting new residents, dealing with their Social Security Disability benefits, and performing a variety of other job duties and responsibilities. As I recall, she used to work for the Federal Social Security Administration and possessed a great deal of knowledge about how to help residents obtain additional benefits. She provided me with a great deal of assistance when Betsy moved into Evergreen Court in 2008. Overall, she was a very good person and support person for Betsy and for me.

During the years that Betsy was a resident, I was never able to learn a great deal about the organizational structure of the facility, other than some of the employees' job duties. There was the general manager, assistant manager, social worker, head chef, kitchen staff, dining room servers and bus staff, home health aides, certified nursing assistants, front desk receptionists, and cleaning staff. Additionally, there were contract nurses and doctors and a medication technologist, who administered the residents' medications.

The social worker who worked at Evergreen Court for many years, (whose name I have forgotten) did his best to assist Betsy by getting her into off-site programs and having her run some of the group counseling sessions. When he retired, there was a gap. After he retired, the social workers came and went. In other words, the turnover was constant. The same applied to the activities director. Overall, I felt that the facility could have been managed better.

I got to know all the receptionists, some of whom had worked there for several years. They were all very nice, competent, and liked Betsy very much. They took messages, transferred calls, handled the patients' mail, managed deliveries and always called me when she was going to the hospital. Overall, it appeared that they were more in charge of managing what was going on than the management staff, whom I rarely saw. There was turnover in the director of the facility (a.k.a. general manager), and the best person I had interacted with left after a few years for a better-paying job.

The weekly menu and activities were posted on a bulletin board. Occasionally some improvements were made to the facility, such as new linoleum flooring to replace the old carpet, repair of some of the residents' bathrooms, and some new carpeting. However, instead of spending money on comfortable couches to replace the very old and torn couches, the owner, Mr. Schonberger, received a donation of several old wooden chairs from some governmental facility. Those chairs were not very comfortable, and the other ones were cheap plastic chairs. I felt bad for the residents because so many of them spent most of the day in the living room which was located near the front reception desk. The living room was neither plush nor comfortable. An antiquated pay phone hung on the wall by the reception desk.

Based on my knowledge, the funding for the owner's facilities came from Social Security Disability at the federal and state levels.

On several occasions I dined with Betsy in the resident dining hall, and I thought that the food was average. Only kosher meals were served, and sometimes the food tasted bland. The residents were assigned to sit at certain tables and generally appeared to be happy. Once in a while, someone would start yelling or screaming, but I never observed any altercations between the residents. Most of them knew each other, and they spent time in small groups. Every resident I met there was very friendly and pleasant, and some of them smiled or laughed.

The dining room had many round tables, comfortable chairs, and carpeting. It was a bit dated but clean and fairly well lit, and there were different places on the first floor where the residents could watch television. In front of the building, there were a few benches for the residents to sit on but not enough to accommodate everyone. During the spring and summer, some of them lay on the grass.

Because the owners had purchased another facility, the Belvedere in Brooklyn, New York (as I recall, sometime around 2015 or later), many services were being cut back at Evergreen Court. My sister, her boyfriend, Frank, and the other residents were very unhappy. I asked Betsy, "Which services?" She noted that the bus had been taken to the NYC facility, vacant positions were not being filled, the food selection had been reduced, etcetera. I asked her how she and her friends were able to go shopping, and she stated, "We have to pool our resources and take a cab." I was shocked and saddened, given that most of the residents had very little, if any, extra spending money.

On a scale from one to ten, I would say that Evergreen Court was a five; the residents were lucky to live there and live safely. I never heard about any criminal activity or fights that required the police to be called.

In March in New York, it is very cold. I imagined that the poor residents—most of whom must have been sleeping at 1:30 a.m., the official time the fire started—had to leave with only the clothes on their backs. I knew that my sister had just been moved to the first floor, as she had a history of falling, and I wondered if she had made it out alone or if she had been assisted by one of the good Samaritans who lived across the street or a firefighter. I imagined all the disabled residents trying to get on the small elevators or climbing down the very narrow and steep stairs to get out.

Fire Photographs
I include many pictures of the fire to present its extent and

severity. Also, to me it was extremely tragic because the residents were disabled and poor people with limited resources. Based on what Betsy and many of them told me about their financial situations, they did not have enough money to buy cigarettes or toiletries or to go shopping for other items. And now, because of the devastating fire, they were all traumatized. They had lost the home they had lived in for many years and had lost all their belongings.

The pictures that follow do not appear in chronological order, and I do not know how many photographers were on the scene.

I want the readers of this book to understand the residents' plight. Moreover, you will read about what happened to my sister shortly after she was sent to the Belvedere and what a terrible downward spiral her life took until her death on September 4, 2022.

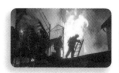 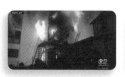 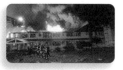

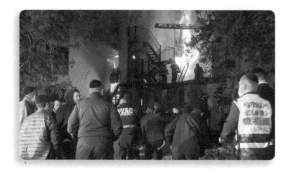

More Online Research about the Fire and More Photographs

When I did a Google search, I reviewed well over one hundred photos. Instead of chronological order, I organized the pictures from the largest flames to what appeared to be the start of the salvage-and-overhaul process. Also included are pictures of the rabbis, one of whom caused the fire.

The Spring Valley firefighters were part of a crew sent into the inferno on March 23, 2021, in hopes of rescuing residents. Lloyd was among the first on the scene.

But at some point, Cich lost track of Lloyd. And, at some point, a section of the Lafayette Avenue building collapsed.

"One minute I was with him the next I wasn't," Cich said. "Somehow we got separated in a matter of feet. I still don't know what happened to this day. We were working to remove the final resident from the building. It's surreal to think." It's been one year since Lloyd, a 35-year-old single father of two young sons, died while he and his fellow firefighters evacuated 112 residents. One resident, 79-year-old Oliver Hueston, died.[21]

After reading more online clips, I learned:

21. M. Castelluccio, "'You Want to See Him Again': 1 Year after Evergreen Court Fire, Lloyd's Loss, Questions Linger," Preserve Ramapo, March 23, 2022, https://preserve-ramapo.com/you-want-to-see-him-again-1-year-after-evergreen-court-fire-lloyds-loss-questions-linger/.

Firefighters spent the overnight hours battling a massive blaze at an assisted living facility in Rockland County. The fire broke out around 1:30 a.m. at the Evergreen Court Home for Adults on Lafayette Street in Spring Valley. On March 23, Lloyd, a 35-year-old Spring Valley firefighter, died when parts of Evergreen Court collapsed as he helped rescue residents of the facility of Lafayette Street. Oliver Hueston, a 79-year-old resident, also died in the inferno.[22]

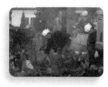
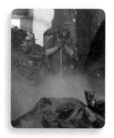

It took over one hundred firefighters from Rockland County to extinguish the fire, and volunteer firefighter Jared Lloyd, whose wife had just given birth to a baby, died on one of the upper floors. Lloyd, who later succumbed to the fire, had yelled, "Mayday!" and then the building fell. I felt sick to my stomach and the most horrified I had ever been about a situation in my life. My mind was racing, and one of my thoughts was that the fire may have been deliberately set so the owners could get the insurance money. I tried hard to dismiss this crude and corrupt possibility. The building was over one hundred years old and was in bad need of upgrades and repairs, although it was not a dump.

22. Steve Lieberman, "Spring Valley Fire: Two Building Inspectors among 6 Charged; Two Accused of Manslaughter," last updated June 30, 2021, lohud.com, https://www.lohud.com/story/news/local/rockland/spring-valley/2021/06/29/spring-valley-fatal-fire-jared-lloyd-arrests-evergreen-adult-home/7797603002/.

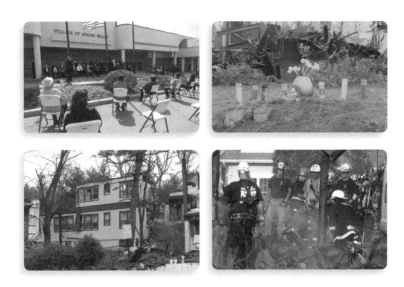

The entire building had burned to the ground, and I realized that my sister and all the residents lost all their belongings, including warm winter clothes.

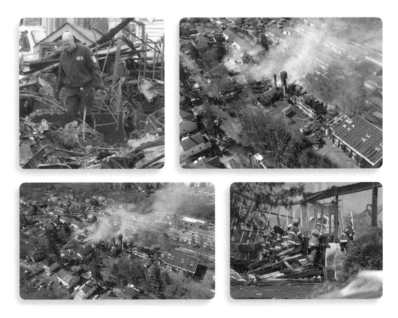

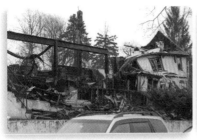
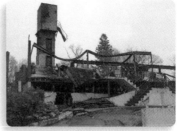

Back to the Phone Call on March 24, 2021, and My Actions

I continued to pedal, and my feet started moving faster out of nervousness and worry. I opened my cell phone and did a quick Google search by typing in "Evergreen Court fire." I was stunned and frightened for Betsy. I do not know what happened to my mind, but I spent a great deal of time, perhaps hours, looking at the videos and photos of the fire. Given the number of pictures (several hundred had already been posted online), I surmised that many fire departments from Rockland and surrounding counties were on site. What I saw horrified me.

On March 24, the day after the fire and the same day Nancy called me, I found the phone number for the Belvedere in Brooklyn, New York, and called to ask about my sister, but was unsuccessful. The phone rang, and rang, and rang, and when I finally got through on that day and over the next few days, I was repeatedly told that my sister was not in her room. It was obvious to me that the officials were more focused on damage control than the need for residents' family members to speak with their loved ones.

On this same day after finishing my exercise on my stationary bike, I wiped my brow and was sipping the last water in my water bottle when the phone rang again. It was a woman with the State of New York, and I immediately thought, "Wow, how wonderful that State of New York officials are already taking charge of the situation, less than twenty-four hours after the fire!" The woman's name was Joan, and she was extremely helpful and understanding. She indicated the main reason for her call was to advise me that the staff from the State of New York were already working on finding placements for the people who had survived the fire. She provided me with access to a listing of all the assisted living facilities throughout the state of New York, so that I could make calls and do research to find a place where my sister could go. I was so happy and knew immediately that Betsy would not be moving to another of the Schonberger family's facilities.

I had previously met the owner of the facility, Mr. Schonberger, who also owned other facilities, but I had no way to contact him. Of course, I wanted to know more about what happened, but over the next few months, I had great difficulty getting through to anyone on the phone, and the general manager at the Brooklyn, New York, facility never returned my calls.

Made Many Phone Calls and Conducted More Research about the Fire: March 5, 2021, to January 2023

While continuing my futile phone calls to reach my sister at the Belvedere in Brooklyn, New York, I conducted more research. My eyes were glued to the computer screen, and I was reminded that the fire was caused by a rabbi who was cleaning the ovens and kitchen at Evergreen Court with a blow torch and a twenty-pound tank in preparation for the Passover dinner and forgot to turn the fire sprinklers back on. I thought, "Are you kidding? He forgot to turn the fire sprinklers back on after he finished cleaning the ovens?"

> The fire erupted after Rabbi Sommer finished cleansing the facility's kitchen and ovens for the Passover holiday with a blowtorch with a twenty-pound propane tank. The building caught fire after they left to cleanse the ovens and kitchen at Golden Acres.[23]

What follows next is a chronology of the news articles I found online starting on March 24, 2021, and ending on January 23, 2023. Please note that there are several-month gaps between the articles, and each time I looked, the order seemed to have changed.

On or around April 2, 2021, I learned that two people who had set the place afire had been arrested, and one of the administrators, Denise Kerr, had also been arrested. But I felt that the saddest fact was that the facility had been cited by the state OSHA board for safety violations, which they may not have corrected. Of course, I had no idea if those safety violations had anything to do with the fire, but a rabbi's incompetence did.

---

23. Steve Lieberman, "Evergreen Court Fire Victim's Sons Sue Facility, Others over His Death. What to Know," last updated November 25, 2022, lohud.com, https://www.lohud.com/story/news/local/rock-land/2022/11/23/evergreen-court-fire-lawsuit-sons-sue-facility-others-over-death/69674055007/.

A seventy-nine-year-old man, Oliver Hueston, who left behind three sons, died in the inferno, and his sons filed a lawsuit against the facility and the employees who were charged in relation to his death. I am not aware of the date of the lawsuit, but the complaint was that the adult home and employees caused Oliver Hueston's death through recklessness and negligence and because staff were poorly trained. Their names were not listed. The sons were seeking a financial award, including punitive damages and legal fees, for their father's death and for the emotional and psychological pain. Their lawsuit named Denise Kerr on the grounds that she hired the father and son rabbis, Nathaniel and Aaron Sommer, to cleanse the facility, even though prosecutors claimed she knew the rabbis lacked the proper permits and failed to take proper precautions. Additionally, the complaint also stated that she was responsible for the training and supervising of the Sommers as well as another former employee, Emanuel Lema.

As of February 2, 2023, prosecutors resolved the cases against the two former Evergreen Green Court employees, adult home director Denise Kerr and worker Manual Lema. Both received adjournments contemplating dismissal and testified before the grand jury.

Lawsuits and Criminal Indictments of Two Rabbis

The mother of the New York firefighter who died in the assisted living facility fire in 2021, Sabrail Davenport, filed a wrongful death suit against the facility, its owners, two contractors, and the village where the fire occurred.

According to the *Journal News*, on September 15, 2022, a Rockland County Court judge upheld the felony indictment against two rabbis linked to the fire. The two rabbis are Nathaniel Sommer and his son, Aaron, who were charged with manslaughter, criminally negligent homicide, reckless endangerment, arson, and assault.

A later article stated:

> A plea may be in the works for the two Rabbis charged in connection with the fatal fire at the Evergreen Court Home for Adults in Spring Valley nearly two years ago that took the life of a resident of the home and a volunteer Spring Valley firefighter. Jared Lloyd's mother, Sabrail Davenport, called "Who Wants to be a volunteer" on Friday, and said she was in court last week, and said she hopes the two defendants, Rabbi Nathaniel Sommer and his son Rabbi Aaron Sommer, aren't treated lightly.

A third lawsuit was filed by Sabrail Davenport over the firefighter's death, alleging negligence and wrongful death against all defendants. On February 3, 2022, she filed a petition to allow the late filing of her claim against the Village of Spring Valley, and on July 15, 2022, she sued the New York State Division of Homeland Security and Emergency Services, seeking to obtain public records pertinent to the fire.

Also, Colin and David Hueston, whose seventy-nine-year-old

father died in the blaze, filed a lawsuit on November 11, 2022, in the State Supreme Court in New York City. The Huestons' lawyers say the lawsuit names the Evergreen Court adult home, including its owners; Rabbi Nathaniel Sommer and his son, Rabbi Aaron Sommer; Evergreen Court director Denise Kerr; and former employee Emmanuel Lema.

Continued Attempts to Speak to My Sister: March 26 to April 2, 2021

Because I care for my husband and had a busy teaching schedule at Florida Atlantic University's College of Business, I could not change plans at the last minute; I was unable to fly to New York. It was an emotional and painful time for me, with Betsy's safety always on my mind. It took me more than one week to get to speak to my sister, and in the meantime, I had no idea how she was feeling, whether she had been hurt, or whether she had shoes and warm clothes. The facility manager or their designee is required to notify the family member about the status of the individual if they have to be sent to a hospital, have fallen, or if there is any other major problem, etcetera. The fact that the only call I received from Nancy, who was not working in the Belvedere facility (she told me this) was to tell me my sister had made it out of the building illustrates the sheer incompetence of the owner of Evergreen Court and the Belvedere. The lack of concern, follow-up, and efficiency of the staff who answered the phone was sickening. Also, whenever I called to leave a message for my sister she never called me back nor did the administrator. However, I was quite certain that the owner, Mr. Schoenberg had provided minimal staffing to save money.

Back to the relentless attempts to speak to my poor sister. First, the different people answering the reception area phone at the Belvedere appeared to not care about who was on the other end, nor what they were inquiring about. They were fast to transfer the phone to someone else or to put you on hold for many minutes. Based on my many years dealing with the staff who worked at the reception desk at Evergreen Court, there was always someone on duty at the front reception desk to answer the phone, twenty-four seven. I knew that employees at Evergreen Court had to work two to three different jobs to live, so I tried to be patient with the staff at the Belvedere. Also, Evergreen Court had constant staff turnover for reasons other than low wages.

When I was finally able to talk to my sister, she could barely speak. She seemed to be in a zombielike state, and I had no idea why. Furthermore, I was unable to find out what, if anything, had happened to her after she was taken out of the burning building, even though on several occasions I attempted to reach a doctor or nurse. Betsy said she was lying in a room that she was confined to, had no clothing except some pants, had lost everything, hadn't seen anybody she knew, was either hot or cold, and hadn't eaten much. When I asked her about the fire, she said she didn't remember a thing about any fire. Her speech was unintelligible, she wasn't in much of a mood to talk, and she wasn't feeling well, so I told her I'd call her back after I obtained more information. I surmised that she was in shock. Once again, partially experiencing and living Betsy's lived experience, I was very worried, sad, shaking, and almost in a state of shock. From the first day, when I had looked at all the pictures, I dreamed about the fire every night for several months.

Of course, I did my best to carry on with my work and care for and be with my dear, loyal, and always supportive husband. I also spent many hours a day on the phone, reviewing online information, and working hard to find a better place for Betsy to live. Below is a list of the facilities I called in New York. I include this information so you can understand the effort and commitment it takes to care for a mentally ill loved one.

List of facilities in different counties and towns in New York:

- The Plaza at Clover
- The Fountains at Riverview
- The Country House in Westchester
- Claremont Village ALP
- Westchester Center for Independent and Assisted Living
- Hedgewood Assisted Living LLC

I wanted her out of downtown NYC and far away from the Schonberger family and their facilities, but I also knew that moving her to Florida was not an option at that time.

Maimonides Medical Center, Brooklyn, New York

A week or so after Betsy had moved to the Belvedere, I was fast asleep when my cell phone rang. I saw that it was 12:30 a.m. and answered it. The caller was a psychiatrist who worked at the Maimonides Medical Center in downtown Brooklyn.

She said, "This is the phone number we were given to call the next of kin." I acknowledged that I was Betsy's sister. The psychiatrist proceeded to tell me that she had no information about Betsy other than that she was dropped off at the emergency room and was completely disoriented and incoherent. She was unable to tell me anything more. I could not find out who had dropped her off at the emergency room, but in my years of interacting with the reception staff at Evergreen Court, someone always called me before Betsy was taken to a hospital by an ambulance.

I said to the psychiatrist, "I don't understand. How could this be?"

She said, "Well, she just was dropped off in the emergency room, and she came in here, and nobody knew anything about her except that she came from some facility in Brooklyn, so I have no information whatsoever about your sister." Shaking, sick to my stomach, almost in tears, and trying to maintain my composure, I told her as much as I could about what had happened to Betsy and where she was currently living. The doctor said, "She is probably in shock, and now that I know about the fire, that makes some sense as to her disorientation." I provided her with additional information about Betsy's background and noted that she had not been hospitalized in the past six or more years for a bipolar episode. The psychiatrist said they would keep her in the hospital for a few more days to see how she was doing. I recapped that I was unable to speak to a doctor about her condition.

Before speaking with the psychiatrist, I had spent several hours researching different facilities in New York and had found a tentative place for Betsy to move to but had not yet completed any paperwork. Less than one day after I spoke to the psychiatrist, I called the Hedgewood ACLF before the end of the workday and told them my sister would not be moving there as tentatively planned because she was in the hospital in Brooklyn. I told them I would get back with them and that I doubted I would approve of her moving there.

Betsy's Illegal Transfer to Hedgewood Assisted Living Facility—Beacon, New York

The next day I attempted several times to reach my sister by phone at the hospital and at the Belvedere, but no one returned my calls. I did not know that she had been transferred to the Hedgewood ACLF in Beacon, New York. On the same day at around 4:30 p.m., I received a phone message from the person in charge of housing at the Hedgewood, and she stated, "Betsy has just arrived here; she is really out of it and appears to be seriously dehydrated." No one gave her any water to drink during the two-and-a-half-hour ride to the Hedgewood ACLF in Beacon, Dutchess County, New York.

The caller continued, "We will find her something to eat, but the cafeteria is already closed for the day. She is very thin, but we will take care of her." Once again, I was horrified, disgusted, sad, and anxious. I strongly felt that the staff of the Hedgewood

Assisted Living Facility received my phone call but had decided to ignore it so that the owner would receive a new resident and their Social Security Disability funds (I have not provided their name to protect their confidentiality).

Betsy's transfer to the facility without my approval and signatures on the legally required forms was a violation of my and my sister's rights under New York State law. I never received any signed forms.

When I again spoke with Nita (the woman in charge of housing) and her boss, the owner, Gail, they both denied receiving any phone call from me and said that I had approved the move, but when I asked for proof, they did not fax or email me anything. Gail was extremely abrasive and was adamant that I had given them permission. She stuck to her story, even after I told her I was my sister's payee for her Social Security Disability benefit, and she told me she did not like the way I was talking to her. When I pushed her about the alleged signed documents, she said that she did not have to give me anything. I hung up on her. What Gail did not know was that because of my expert witness work I had a great deal of knowledge about factual evidence; in this case, without documents containing my signature, I hadn't approved anything.

I was fuming, and once again my mind was racing because I was very afraid for and worried about my sister. They said they would keep her there until I came to pick her up and told me that they would not pay to have a medevac transport her to another facility. How patientcare oriented they were not!

The next day I called the New York State Department of Health and filed complaints with the complaint center. I felt very lucky that one of the directors, Anthony, returned my call. I include one of the letters they sent to me to demonstrate that government officials do respond to your complaints.

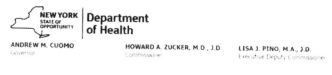

NEW YORK STATE OF OPPORTUNITY

Department of Health

ANDREW M. CUOMO
Governor

HOWARD A. ZUCKER, M.D., J.D.
Commissioner

LISA J. PINO, M.A., J.D.
Executive Deputy Commissioner

April 21, 2021

Linsey Willis
779 St. Albans Drive
Boca Raton, FL 33486

Re: The Belvedere
5110 19th Avenue
Brooklyn, NY 11204
Complaint Case #: NY00274948

Dear Ms. Willis:

This letter is to acknowledge receipt of your complaint filed through the N.Y.S. Department of Health Adult Home Complaint Hotline on April 21, 2021. The name of the facility and assigned case number are listed above.

The investigator assigned to your complaint may contact you for further information. If you have questions about the complaint status, please contact the Metropolitan Area Regional Office at (212) 417-4440.

The investigation of your complaint will be done according to the Regional Office's schedule and therefore we ask you to allow the surveyor sufficient time to perform the investigation prior to calling for a status update. Once the Regional Office completes the investigation they will advise you of the results.

Sincerely,

Michael Rinaldi

Michael Rinaldi
Statewide Complaint Manager
Office of Primary Care and Health Systems Management

Empire State Plaza, Corning Tower, Albany, NY 12237 | health.ny.gov

During the first sixteen years of my career, I worked for several government agencies, and I know that many people do not view government employees in a positive light. For example, many people view those who work for the government as faceless, incompetent, and lazy bureaucrats. There are competent and incompetent employees working in the public and private sectors.

One of the top administrators with the agency, Anthony, even took the time to return my call. We had a very productive discussion, and I carefully summarized for him what had transpired at Evergreen Court, the Belvedere, and Hedgewood, where my sister was living. I told him that she had been sent there without my permission.

I called the Belvedere, was finally able to reach Nancy (the woman who used to work for Evergreen Court and whose last name I have left out to protect her privacy), whom the staff had transferred me to, even though she was not working at the Belvedere. She told me that there was paperwork, and I should ask the owner of the facility Betsy was transferred to. She had no other information, nor did anyone at the front desk, though they should have been able to tell me when Betsy left the hospital, when she was picked up by a medevac, and what time she was shipped to upstate New York. Once again, I could not obtain any useful information.

Care Packages for Betsy and Other Survivors

One of the ways I coped with my shock and sadness about the fire at Evergreen Court was to make a plan for sending clothing and shoes to the survivors, many of whom I knew. I realized before I started that this was not going to be an easy task, given the length of time it took me to be able to speak to Betsy, but I was fully committed to calling and speaking with as many people as possible. I found out that fifty-two of the survivors were sent to the Belvedere (one of the facilities owned by the Schonberger family), but I knew that it would be next to impossible to talk to everyone. I started the process after finalizing where Betsy was going to move. I felt terrible that everyone had lost all their belongings and that most of them would have to live at the Belvedere, and I wanted to help.

On April 2, 2021, I called the reception desk at the Belvedere, and I asked to be transferred to the day room, where the residents socialized. When someone answered the phone, I introduced myself, asked them if they remembered me, and said that I wanted to help them. Most of them knew me and Betsy; some of them told me that they were her friend and asked about her because they had not seen her around that facility. Their first names were Mitch, Frank, Edward, two Alices, Sandra, Velma, and Phillip. I was unable to speak to anyone else and was so happy that each person was willing to talk to me. My strategy was to start with the first person, ask them to pass me on to the next person in the day room, and so on. After several calls I was able to speak to all the people I mentioned.

I asked them how they were feeling and what clothing they needed. Each person gave me specific details about the piece of clothing they needed the most. I jotted everything down, including their shoe size, waist size, etc. They were elated and so happy that someone cared enough to call and ask about them.

Considering what they had been through and how they were feeling, I felt that I had accomplished a great deal. I made sure each person knew that they would be receiving a care package wrapped in brown paper with their names boldly written on it with a marker pen. This was an important detail because I knew the box would be delivered via UPS to the front reception desk, be opened, and then each resident would be notified that they had mail.

The next steps in my plan were to go shopping at the local Goodwill store and then empty out my closet for older clothes for Betsy. When I told two of my friends what I was doing, they wanted to lend a hand. My friend and associate Bob went through his closet and brought me a few boxes of pants and tops. He is a tall man and had lost weight, so the sizes could be used by more than one man. I went to my friend Diane's house, and we went through her mother's clothes. Her mother had just passed away, and I was so elated and thankful that she invited me to come over and go through everything. When she told her husband, Bill, about what we were doing, he went to his closet and gathered up some clothes.

I thanked Bob, Diane, and Bill for their generosity and interest in contributing to my cause.

The next step was to sort all the clothes on my dining room table by male, female, type, and size. I had already purchased the boxes and brown wrapping paper and started assembling the packages. When I finished wrapping, labeling, and marking each package, the largest box was prepared for shipping via UPS to the Belvedere. The smaller box was prepared for shipping to Green Hills Estates, the place I had selected for my sister to move to. I was so happy that the box would be in her room when she arrived.

I did worry whether the boxes would get lost, and my worst-case scenario thought was, "What if the residents and Betsy never receive their packages?" These thoughts were negative, but given my experience with the staff at the Belvedere, I had reason to be concerned. Because I was distrustful of the staff at the Belvedere and the Schonberger, I called the facility a few days later and was told that the box had arrived. However, when I called the residents to find out whether they received their packages, only one person had received his. When I called back again to track down where the packages went, I was told they had been taken to another one of the Schonberger's facilities. My mouth was hanging open, my eyes were rolling, and my head was shaking. I was disgusted but not surprised. At this point I decided that I was not going to take the time to find out whether the box could be returned to the Belvedere. It would have been a waste of time and energy to do this. The only positive outcome was that my sister's box arrived at Green Hills Estates, and I was told that the box had been placed in her room. I took a deep breath in and breathed out.

Betsy's Move to Green Hills Estates, Haverstraw, New York, on or around April 7, 2021

I was finally able to settle on a place in Haverstraw, New York—Green Hills Estates.

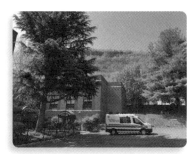 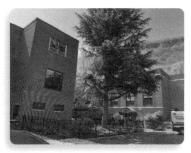

Fortunately, one of the nurses there knew my sister, and the contract doctors did, as well. I finally felt a bit more comfortable about her new home. I also saw pictures of the facility and spoke to several people, including one of the owners, Mr. Sanchez.

On or around April 7, 2021, I booked a flight, hotel, and rental car and flew to New Jersey. The main purpose of the trip was to pick Betsy up at the Hedgewood Facility and drive her to her new home. Of course, Murphy's Law intervened when I least expected it and when it was least needed. When I arrived at the car rental counter in Newark, there were some problems, and when I finally left for Hedgewood, I hadn't eaten anything in over five hours and was existing only on adrenaline.

Driving out of Newark is a horror scene, particularly when you are hungry, tired, upset, and worried. I drove out of the Newark Airport not knowing how bad the traffic was going to be or that I would be diverted off my route. As many of you may have experienced, when you drive using the mapping apps on your phone, some work better than others. Well, Murphy's Law continued to plague me, as I got off at the wrong exit and ended up in a scary neighborhood with an inordinate number of cars parked all over the road. It was starting to rain. I got out of there as quickly as possible.

I passed Haverstraw, New York, where Betsy was going to be living, and I made my way along the main road through the Hudson Valley, which crossed from one side to the other of the Hudson River. The rain continued as the evening darkness descended, and I was a nervous, hungry, and distraught wreck. As I was driving in the dark, I crossed a very narrow bridge to the other side of the Hudson River, and when I looked to my right and up, I saw a high mountain and was worried and nervous that I was lost.

The time was about 5:30 p.m., and as Murphy's Law continued to affect my trip, I started to panic. I have always hated getting lost or feeling lost, and this time I was scared. I started breathing very heavily, and for the first time in my life, I felt like I was about to have a nervous breakdown. After crossing a very narrow bridge back to the west side of the Hudson River, I immediately pulled over to the side of the road, took a deep breath, and started to weep. My body was shaking, and I continued to breath harder and at a rapid pace.

My father used to tell me that he would say, "This, too, shall pass," while he served on a navy destroyer during WWII; he would also tell me "This, too, shall pass," to calm me down. I picked up the phone, and I called the Hedgewood ACLF, and the woman who answered told me that I was almost there. I was not lost and was only five minutes away.

I stopped crying, swallowed, wiped my brow, and drove on. When I arrived, the woman was helping my sister walk to the car. Betsy was carrying a medium-sized, black, plastic garbage bag and was wearing torn slippers. She was extremely disheveled and gaunt, looking like skin and bones. I thanked the woman, who apologized for the confusion and reiterated that they never received the call. I said, "Let's not discuss that again, because it's over." She was not the one at fault, because she was not the owner. Being a conscientious employee, she indicated that I would have to pay them for the few days my sister was there, and I assured her I would send her a check. When I returned home, I mailed them a check.

Betsy looked older than I'd ever seen her look before and was weak and barely able to speak. I was very worried that she might be in the process of dying. I learned later that my fears were accurate. As stressed and upset as I was, I was so glad to be there for her, even though I had suffered along the way. While driving to Haverstraw in the pitch-black dark, I tried to start a conversation with Betsy but didn't receive much response, other than that she was tired and hungry and didn't care where she was going. I told her that she would like where she would be living and that she would have her own room on a newly renovated floor of the facility.

When we arrived at Green Hills Estates in Haverstraw, New York, it was evening, and I was greeted by some of the staff, who escorted us to the second floor and took her to her room. The floor looked like a hospital ward, but it was extremely clean, there was a large closet, a chest of drawers, and a comfortable chair; the rooms were large, and all the furniture was brand new. In the hallway, there was a long and spacious nurse's desk, and nearby were six large, really nice leather chairs and a very large flat-screen TV.

In summary, Green Hills Estates was very different from what she had at Evergreen Court, because the building there was well over a hundred years old and the owners were not keeping the place up as they should have. While I was at Green Hills Estates, I met a few people who had lived at Evergreen Court before the fire and knew Betsy. She did not seem to care. I did not recognize the signs of the beginning of her death.

In Person Visit to Obtain Refund and Business Ethics

Everyone who owns a business and serves the public should act in an ethical manner. There is a great deal of literature about ethical principles and practices and how to deal with people who are behaving in an unethical manner. I know this because for the twenty-five years I was a college instructor, there was always a section on ethics in the textbooks I used.

Based on my experience and knowledge of how the Schonberger family managed their business at Evergreen Court, I know they were unethical, ineffective, and inefficient managers. They were poor leaders and were primarily focused on money. The following section of this chapter is about what I experienced and ended up having to do after the fire to receive a refund check from the owners. If I had not put forth the effort to obtain the money the Schonbergers owed me, I would have never been reimbursed.

I waited about a month after the fire to contact the accounting office for Evergreen Court, which was located in New Jersey. To be courteous and understanding, I did not contact them immediately, because they all probably needed time to process what had happened during and after the fire. However, I called numerous times to speak to someone on the telephone, and each time the mailboxes for all staff were full, or no one answered the phone. I finally decided to send a certified letter (see next page) and included a copy of the check voucher (see following pages), but sending the letter and documentation made absolutely no difference to the staff working in the office.

It made no difference that I included proof, because the certified letter and numerous calls over the next several months did not result in any responsible action on their part. Not only was I upset about my sister's plight, but I was also dealing with a group of unethical people. I say "group" because I left messages with several people besides Raidy (see letter) when the various mailboxes were not full.

Linsey C. Willis
779 Saint Albans Drive
Boca Raton, FL 33486

Attn: Raidy
Evergreen Court Accounting Office
1770 West County Line Road
Suite 102
Lakewood, NJ 08701

June 3, 2021

Dear Raidy,

Thank you for taking my call on 6/1/21. As per our conversation enclosed are the documents which were completed regarding my sister, Betsy Craig. The documents are; 1) a copy of the proof of payment (i.e., check voucher) for the security deposit I was required to provide before she moved into Evergreen Court; 2) Admission Agreement (which I was never provided with a signed copy for); and the Evergreen Court Retirement Residence agreement.

FYI, I have am my sister's payee, Power of Attorney and Advanced Medical Directive representative.

Please provide me with a check made out to Linsey C. Willis in the amount of $2,375.96 at your earliest possible convenience.

Also, FYI, my sister no longer resides in one of the Schaumberger's (I hope I spelled their name correctly) facilities. She is a survivor of the fire that destroyed Evergreen Court which occurred on or around March 23, 2021.

Thank you and have a safe and happy day.

Linsey C. Willis

Recd. 7/
Fr.

CHECK VOUCHER

Advance Housing, Inc.

VENDOR INFORMATION

VENDOR NAME: Lindsey Willis   VENDOR NUMBER   NEW VENDOR? YES ☒ NO ☐

NAME PAYABLE TO (If different than vendor name): Lindsey Willis (for Betsy Cra...

ADDRESS   CITY   STATE   ZIP: 779 St Albans Dr

TELEPHONE   Boca Raton Fl 33486

SPECIAL INSTRUCTIONS

Give Check to Danda + f live mail out —

ACCOUNT INFORMATION

ACCOUNT DESCRIPTION	EXPENSE ACCOUNT NUMBER	COST CENTER	AMOUNT
Acct	Betsy Craig (004)		$2,375.96
Closing out Betsy Craig	personal money — closed as of 6/1/08		
	2800-004		

INVOICE INFORMATION

INVOICE NUMBER	INVOICE DUE DATE	CHECK NUMBER	CHECK DATE	INVOICE AMOUNT

Prepared by: L Crk   Date: 7/18/08   Chief Financial Officer   CEO/President

When I was finally able to speak to Raidy, on two occasions she told me that the check was being sent. This was not true, and I knew then that the management staff of Schonberger's company was never going to send me the money. My only choice was to take a trip to New Jersey, visit my friends Alan and Brenda, and then go visit Betsy. I strongly felt that if I showed up in person, I would receive the check, and was looking forward to using the money for Betsy's needs. By this time it had been six months since I sent the letter.

When I provided Brenda with the address of the accounting office, she laughed, because it was in the New Jersey town where she grew up. In fact, she knew exactly where the office building was located. Our husbands, Alan and Frank, wished us luck but believed that I would be unsuccessful in obtaining a check for the money I was owed. I told them I would get the money. When I set my mind on completing a goal and the tasks involved in doing so, I am usually successful.

We decided to make a surprise visit, because if they knew I was coming, they would not come to the office door or would lock it. I felt that this would happen because of what had previously transpired. The office building was about twelve miles from Brenda and Alan's home in New Jersey. We went into the office lobby, which was very small and cramped, and saw that the main door was open. There was no receptionist, so I walked inside and asked if anyone was there. A man got up and walked my way, appearing annoyed that I just walked in, and asked me what I wanted. I explained why I was there and said that I needed to see Raidy. He immediately responded, "She is out of the office," at which point I asked him when she would be back. He said, "Probably after lunch, but I am not sure. I will let her know you came by, and she will send you a check." I immediately told him I was going to wait for the check, because I had flown up from Florida and was not leaving without it. His face became red, and he told me he had just started working there. I then insisted that he call her to advise her of my presence.

I looked around the office area, which had several cubicles and very cheap-looking furniture, and there were no employees sitting at any of the desks. I then asked him if I could speak with the person in charge. He immediately responded, saying, "No one else is here but me." Then I heard some shuffling of papers, looked to my right, and saw an opening, which was apparently another office in the back. I walked that way, and the young man tried to stop me. I was not giving up. I said hello to the man at the desk, and it was quite apparent that he was very upset that I had just walked back there. I told him why I was there and said that I was waiting to receive a check, at which point he used an alibi: "Raidy is not here. She is responsible for writing checks. We will send you a check, or you can come back tomorrow. I cannot help you." It was obvious that he was hoping I would leave. I knew that if Brenda and I left, we would never again gain access to their facility, nor would I ever receive a check. They had no intention of paying me what they owed.

The man who was working in the back office told me to get out of his office and go into the lobby. Not knowing what he planned to do, as I was walking back to the main entrance, I stopped to speak to the man I met when first I walked into the office, and I asked him if he knew about the fire and what happened to the residents. I also told him that my sister was at the Belvedere and that the money they owed me was hers. I also mentioned that I had read that there was an investigation going on about what happened and that lawsuits could be filed. I knew this comment would result in a reaction from the man in the back. He was obviously listening to me and immediately came out of his office and walked quickly to where I was standing. He made several angry, loud, and shrill statements: "You are trespassing. If you do not get out now, I am calling the police. You have no right to be here. You have no business talking to him [the other man]. Now get out." As I was backing out of the door, I told him I was waiting for Raidy to return. Then I sat down in the chair next to Brenda, and he slammed and locked the door. However, I do not think he knew that I was not leaving, nor who he was dealing with. I was not going anywhere. While we sat there, I could hear that he was making a phone call, and I believe there were two reasons I heard him. The walls were paper thin, and he was worried. He was calling his boss and did not know what to do about me. Brenda and I laughed at his behavior.

A few minutes later, he opened the door and said he had spoken with his boss, who was the general manager of the Belvedere in Brooklyn, New York, and that I was to wait for Raidy to return. I knew who he was calling, because I had tried to reach the man on numerous occasions to obtain information about my sister, but he did not bother to return my calls.

Brenda and I waited for about an hour, and before Raidy returned, the man in the back opened the door and again started to yell at me in a shrill voice while he was simultaneously speaking with the man—his boss, the general manager of the Belvedere—on the other end of the phone line. I was so surprised that he was yelling at me that I took his picture. I was almost afraid that he would move my way and slug me. My arrival at the accounting office and my comments had apparently caused them some stress.

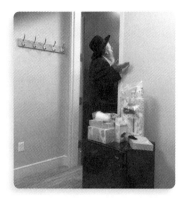

Overall, none of them were happy about my presence, nor were they the least bit customer-service oriented. If they were at all concerned about their customers—in this case, my sister, Betsy—I would not have had to go to their accounting office in person over six months after I had written and mailed them a certified letter, and I would not have pursued the matter in a somewhat aggressive manner.

When Raidy returned, her almost immediate alibi was that she thought the check had been sent and that she would send me the check as soon as possible. The look on her face and her body language made it appear that she was nervous and surprised that I was there in person. I told her I would wait for her to write the check. When I told her I was flying back to Florida, she also looked surprised. We waited about twenty minutes, and she brought me the check. However, the printing was slanted, and it did not look authentic, so I asked her to reprint the check, which she begrudgingly did. Her comment was, "What is wrong with the way it looks? It can still be deposited." When I had the second check in my hand, my immediate thought was that she may have given me a fake check. When I returned home, I immediately deposited it in the bank, because I did not want them to stop payment on it. Unfortunately, I felt this way because of their rude, obstinate and abrasive behavior, which was very unsettling to me.

Regarding business ethics, there are several more very salient points I feel compelled to include, based on my education and years of experience. For example, I have taught management and human resources courses for over twenty-five years (1998 to 2023), completed a several-day ethics training program, conducted several one-week leadership workshops, taught situational leadership, and served as an expert witness on sixty cases across the United States for employment law and personal injury attorneys. I always ask for copies of the organization's policies and procedures, ethics code, and employee handbook. There are many cases where a company and/or government management personnel have violated the written ethics principles and practices. My ending comment is usually, "If the leaders of the organization had acted in an ethical manner and had the moral courage to do the right thing, the situation would have not occurred." The worst case is a lawsuit against the organization. It is ironic that several lawsuits have been filed because of the fire. However, shortly after the fire, I predicted that lawsuits would be filed.

I feel strongly that the degree of effort I had to exercise to receive the $2,375 refund represented unethical behavior. The effort I had to put forth to obtain the refund and the fact that when I showed up in the Schonberger's' accounting office the staff were not only rude, but difficult to deal with, indicated to me that they had no intention of ever sending me a check. Also, I observed and experienced the violations of the State of New

York's laws, poor management and leadership, their failure to act, and a lack of accountability on the part of the owners and staff of the Schonbergers' company, which reflect numerous ethical breaches. Moreover, the following pattern of events (all of which have been discussed in this book) substantiates this statement:

- *failing* to resolve OSHA violations over many years, as documented in various online news articles: "Spring Valley's enforcement of state fire and building codes had become so bad that the state deputized the Rockland County government to take charge in early 2022. A state monitor had been assigned for years to Spring Valley Building Department, as well. While the monitor was at the department, the village went several years not filing the 2013 reports with the state Department of State."[24]

- *reducing* services for the residents of Evergreen Court (based on anecdotal evidence and my observations) shortly after the Schonbergers purchased the Belvedere: the bus services were eliminated because the bus was transferred to the Belvedere; repairs were not completed; staffing was cut back and the quality of meals declined

---

24. Steve Lieberman, "Evergreen Court Fire: Charges against Former Spring Valley Building Inspector Dismissed," *Rockland Westchester Journal News*, February 2, 2023.

- *negligence* on the part of the rabbis who were contracted to prepare the Passover meals, because they forgot to turn the fire alarm on when they finished cleaning the ovens, which was one of the causes of the fire
- *sending* my sister to the Maimonides Medical Center in Brooklyn, New York, without notifying me
- *failing to* return my numerous calls to the Belvedere, by the facility administrator, doctors, and nurses, whom I was calling to find out how my sister was after she was transferred to the facility after the fire
- *allowing* the transfer of my sister to the Hedgewood Assisted Living Facility, which took two and a half hours, during which time she was not provided with any water, resulting in her arrival in a severely dehydrated state
- *referring* me to Nancy, who, at the time, was not working at the Belvedere (and was no longer employed by Evergreen Court because the facility had burned down), to respond to my questions about my sister, when she had no information or official documentation to provide to me
- *telling me*, through Nancy, that the legally required paperwork to transfer my sister to the Hedgewood Assisted Living Facility had been completed and that I had signed it, which was totally untrue
- *taking* the UPS box, which contained individually wrapped and labeled sealed packages with

each person's name affixed, to another of the Schonberger's' facilities instead of delivering the packages to the residents at the Belvedere

In summary, I believe it is possible that, had the management staff of the Schonbergers' properties been effective and ethical managers with leadership skills, none of the aforementioned would have occurred. Of course, the worst of the events was the catastrophic fire, which could have been prevented and which is the primary subject of this chapter.

Last Social Visit with Betsy

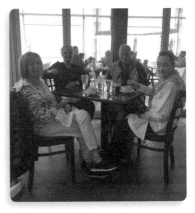

This is a picture of Betsy, my dear friends Brenda and Alan, and me. The week of October 21, 2021, I went to visit Betsy at Green Hills Estates with Brenda and Alan. We picked her up and took her to get her hair cut, and then we all went out for a late lunch. Betsy looked worse than ever before. This lunch was the last time I went out with my sister, and we were blessed to have had that time with Brenda and Alan.

More Hospitals and Rehabilitation Facilities

For almost the entire year after the fire, Betsy spent most of her time in rehabilitation facilities, hospitals, and ICU units of hospitals in and near Nyack, New York. Her placements at these facilities were due to of a variety of ailments, many of which I observed, such as serious dehydration, not being alert, inability to feed herself without help, and inability to walk without a cane and walker. I had not realized that these were indicative of the beginning of dementia. I was also told by the doctors and nurses that she had blood in her stool. The doctor said she could have cancer. They also told me that she needed tactile stimulation and that she had a severe infection (which turned into sepsis), pneumonia, an elevated white blood count, declining kidney function, and COPD. She was not eating and had severe weight loss of over twenty pounds in a three-month period; she was down to 102 pounds. Each time I spoke with a nurse or doctor, I took notes and wrote down the dates but never realized that these were signs leading to dementia and death. I strongly believe that my sister started to die when she was sent to the Maimonides Medical Center in Brooklyn, New York, on April 6, 2021. I strongly believe many of her medical problems were related to the fire. She was in a state of shock, and her mental and physical states began to decline.

During a stay in a local hospital near Haverstraw, New York, on August 15, 2022 (I do not recall the name), a dietician called me and provided me with additional disturbing and very sad news. She told me that Betsy weighed ninety pounds, was confused, was not aware of what she was doing, and was having difficulty swallowing. And then she asked me if Betsy had signed an advanced medical directive that included a do-not-resuscitate order (DNR). I told her that Betsy had one.

I spoke to three different staff members over the next several days, from August 15 to 26. Then, when Betsy returned to Green Hills Estates shortly before her imminent death, the nurses told me that she was exhibiting signs of Alzheimer's. She was disrobing and walking outside her room, hitting residents, and being aggressive. And then I was again asked if my sister had a DNR order. Things were moving too fast, and I finally realized that Betsy not only had serious health conditions, but that she would also soon be an Alzheimer's patient. I prayed for the best but expected the worst, because the two nurses told me that if Betsy did not start to eat on her own, they would have to send her back to the hospital so she could be put on an eating program with a completely different diet, one that was all liquid. Apparently, they were not going to tell me that she was dying. At this point I prayed to God that if it was her time, to please take her and not let her become a vegetable in a hospital bed, because I did not want her to suffer anymore. I also asked God to allow her to live long enough for me to see her. The bottom line was that I would be there for her, no matter when I had to fly up to New York.

GOD WAS THERE 10

Overview

The last week of my sister's life was the most agonizing time of my life since the deaths of my parents in 2006 and 2007. I did not realize that as early as May 2022, she was starting to lose a great deal of weight: twenty-three pounds.

This chapter is probably one of the most important in the book because of what I experienced on my way to see Betsy and what transpired before her death. Those few days will be with me for the rest of my life.

Recap of the Last Few Months of Betsy's Life

As noted previously, during the last several months of Betsy's life, she was in and out of rehabilitation facilities for her trouble walking and other related ailments. She was sent back to the last place she would live, Green Hills Estates in Haverstraw, New York. The hospital is nine miles from Green Hills Estates. As usual, I spent a great deal of time on the phone trying to reach her at the different facilities and was only able to speak to her on a few occasions. About two weeks before she passed away, two nurses at Green Hills Estates told me that the reason she was sent to a nursing home was so they could try to get her to eat and that she was on liquids only. I was asked about a feeding tube, and I did not approve this. I realized then that perhaps she was dying but would not admit it to myself. When the two nurses asked me if I had a signed DNR order from Betsy. Stupidly, I asked why and was told that if she continued to not eat, this could be a problem. A few days later, she was transferred to Nyack Hospital.

Things were moving so fast again, with what was happening to my dear sister. After I spoke by phone to a night-shift doctor at the hospital, I feared the worst. Her life would be ending soon. Even though he called me after 10:30 p.m., I was lucky to speak to him, because it's very difficult to actually have a conversation with a doctor; I was so grateful for the times that I was able to do so regarding my sister's care. Nonetheless, there was never any consistency with which doctor was taking care of my sister at any given time because they work different shifts and/or are contract Drs. After the fire, I was told by different doctors that she had Parkinson's disease, was in and out of attentiveness, and had difficulty speaking. Practically every health care professional identified a different illness or disability. I spoke to several different doctors at Nyack Hospital and Northern Riverview Healthcare Center, in Haverstraw, New York; it was difficult to keep track of everything. Also, because I was upset during each call, sometimes I forgot to take adequate notes.

Late on Sunday night, August 28, 2022, I spoke to the doctor. He advised me that Betsy was not doing well and that she had COPD. This was the first time I had been advised that she was suffering from this. He told me that she had continued to lose weight and that her feeding tube had been removed. I had previously approved removal of the tube. The other horrible facts he stated were, "She is one hundred pounds and is no longer conscious." I told him I was coming to New York on September 9, and he told me, "She will probably not last until then. You need to come as soon as possible." In hindsight, I should have just said, "I will be there ASAP."

The next day, August 29, 2022, I spoke to the palliative care nurse, and we discussed setting up a FaceTime call. She advised me that even if I arrived in the next day or two, my sister might not last that long. My mind was racing and racing, and the tears were streaming. She asked for my approval to take Betsy off all life support and to do a DNR. I approved. I didn't want my sister to linger in a hospital in a vegetative state.

I went about my usual business; I tried to stay strong and positive and did not cancel my two commitments. One was a workshop in Miami, Florida, which I could not cancel because it would have caused problems for the HR department and well over twenty-five employees, but another instructor was able to cover two dates I was scheduled to teach at Florida Atlantic University and other meetings I had. I could not get to New York any earlier than Thursday of that week. I prayed to the Lord that Betsy would wait for me and to give me strength, perseverance, and patience to handle what was coming my way. No matter what happened on my journey to the Newark airport in New Jersey, I knew I could cope. Newark is the best city to fly into to then drive to upstate New York.

The most stressful, most agonizing, and scariest part of my preparations to go to New York was my FaceTime call with the palliative nurse. I left the FIU campus in Miami, Florida, while there was a torrential downpour of rain. I called the nurse back as I was driving, and she encouraged me to go to a stopping place as soon as possible so I could speak to Betsy on FaceTime. I told her that I was driving through almost hurricane-condition rain and could not stop on the turnpike, but she pleaded that I stop as soon as I could. She was greatly concerned that I had to speak with and see Betsy on FaceTime ASAP. She also told me that it did not matter when I arrived in New York, as she might die on my way up; at which point I did my best to not run off the road. Many idiot drivers do not slow down in rainy conditions.

I became increasingly scared that I would not be able to say goodbye to Betsy and again asked God to have her wait for me. I was in a state of shock, fear, great grief, and anxiety, but I kept driving. It was too dangerous to pull over, but about fifteen minutes into the horrific drive, I was able to get off at an exit. I pulled over as far to the right as possible and onto the grass, took a deep breath, because I was in panic mode, dialed the number, and continued to pray.

Betsy was totally uncommunicative because she was unconscious, although her eyes were open. I held the phone very close to my face and talked very loudly into it. I told her I was on my way and that I loved her and asked her to please wait for me. I also apologized for not coming sooner. The nurse (who, by the way, was my guardian angel) told me to ask her to blink if she understood, and she did. God was there.

When I arrived home to Boca Raton, I was distraught and wiped out and felt like a ton of bricks had been dumped on me. I was not even sure whether I could get on the plane the next morning, but after a poor night's sleep, I made it to Nyack, New York, after leaving the Newark airport. My initial plans changed at the last minute because I decided to stay overnight with my dear friends of many years, Brenda and Alan, because I did not want to arrive in Nyack, New York, at night. She drove me to Nyack the next morning, and I visited Betsy. Again, God was there for me.

God blessed me again when the hospital allowed me to stay in her private room in a sleeping chair. I spent about two and a half quality days by her side and only left to eat two meals. I was so elated that I was again there for her during her darkest hours. I had more gratitude, thankfulness, and belief in God than I had ever had before. Betsy waited for me, and we were together one last time.

I blinded myself to the condition of Betsy's skin, bones, face, and her heavy breathing and coped by reading to her. The nurses encouraged me to talk to her as much as I could, to touch her, and to ask her to blink her eyes to let me know she heard me. I was amazed that she did. Whenever I asked her to, she did. She also moved her head, arm, or hand when I touched each one. Her body was still warm. Her legs were wrapped in warm leggings, and although she had no feeding tube, she was being given liquid intravenously, as well as a morphine drip.

I took a picture from where I was sitting because I saw a street sign, "Rotary Way," and I am an active member of the Rotary Club of Downtown Boca Raton in Boca Raton, Florida.

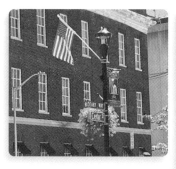
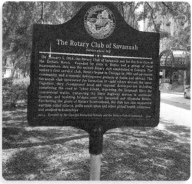

The sign comforted me somewhat, because the Rotary Club is the world's largest service organization, whose members serve others throughout the world. I was serving my sister in her time of greatest need. Several times, I have seen a Rotary Club sign while traveling (e.g., Banff, Alberta, Canada, and Savannah, Georgia).

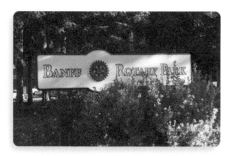

I then walked down the street to a local bookstore and purchased a few books, one I was planning to read to Betsy. On my way back to the hospital, I was lucky enough to receive a phone call from one of my friends from the Rotary Club, Diane Stevens. Speaking with her comforted me.

I bought three books at a local bookstore in the quaint town of Nyack. One of the books, *Outliers*, was by Malcolm Gladwell, and I read almost the entire book to her. Sometimes I read for more than an hour without stopping, sometimes very close to her at her bedside, other times farther away. I would not have missed reading to her for "all the tea in China."

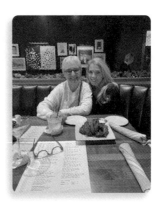

The Last Two and a Half Days of Betsy's Life

While I was sitting very close to my sister's head and face, something very spiritual happened. While looking at her and not thinking anything in particular, these words came out of my mouth: "You will never be forgotten. You are a valuable person and had, at one time, a wonderful life, and I will ensure that you will never be forgotten."

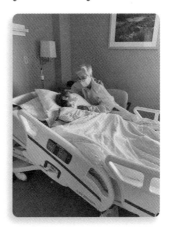

Then I reminded her of the book I had started writing and that she had contributed to. I said that it would be finished and would be a *New York Times* bestseller. I also told her that I wanted people to know who she was at one time, what had happened to her, and how brave she was to have struggled so long with her illness.

In summary, I still do not believe it but am so grateful that the words spilled out of my mouth—"I love you, and you will never be forgotten"—to my dear sister at her deathbed. *God was there.*

I asked the night nurse if it would be okay if I could move the chair into the hallway and of course she granted my request. I could no longer listen to her heavy breathing. She then told me that based on her observations and knowledge many dying patients wait until their loved ones leave the room to take their last breath.

Betsy passed away September 4, 2022, at 4:45 a.m. She was sixty-seven years old. God rest your soul, Betsy!

I watched outside the door as the hospital staff cleaned her body, put it in a bag, and was wheeled to the bed. I took a quick shower and then said goodbye to the staff and made my way to the hospital entrance to hail a Lyft to the train station. I could have taken a cab but enjoyed taking the train to the Newark airport because during each trip I have taken in the past I have time to reflect and relax. It was a gloomy morning and I stood quietly and tried not to cry.

When I arrived at the airport I was directed to the wrong location and while waiting I realized there was a problem with my ticket: I had booked the return for the next day because my friend Diane, who lived in Bethlehem, wanted me to visit she and her husband on my way back to Florida. While standing in the line, I decided to go straight home but was then directed to a different line and another counter. The ticket agent there told me that they would try to get me on a flight the same day. Even though she did not charge me and said everything would be okay, I started to cry.

I did not call Diane until after the ticket change had been made. When I called her she pleaded with me to change my mind and indicated that a visit might do me some good but I told her it was too late and that she and her husband, Bevin, would not enjoy my company. I knew then that I had made the right decision to go straight home and not to Bethlehem, Pennsylvania. I have never been a person to lay my troubles on other people, even long term close friends.

A week or so after learning of my sister's passing, the Rotary Club sent me some beautiful flowers. When I received them, I considered them to be Betsy's flowers.

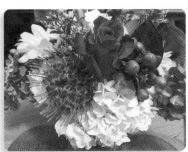

The Quilt

God was in my presence again a few months later. I was reorganizing my linen closet and remembered that Betsy had made me a quilt, which was stored in the guest bedroom closet.

I hadn't thought about, touched, moved, or looked at it for over twenty years. It was enclosed in a thick plastic bag. I reached up and removed it from

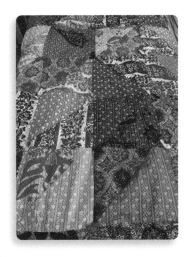

the metal pull-out basket, took it to my bedroom, and spread it out on my bed. My husband was in the bedroom, and when he looked at the quilt, he noted how gorgeous it was and that he was very impressed that Betsy had made it by hand and without a sewing machine.

We decided to place the quilt at the foot of our bed on the wooden bench. It even matched two sets of new sheets. After placing it at the foot of our bed, I was almost in tears and thought that Betsy had facilitated this from heaven. She wanted me to make use of the best gift she had ever given me. She made it for me while I was in college.

I believe that Betsy's spirit is present in the quilt and that she was happy I had removed it from the closet. *God was there.*

Postscript

I called a few attorneys in New York, and no one would take the case because they said: my sister did not earn any money, her death was not close enough to the date of the fire, and/or I would have to obtain medical records from the time of the fire to her death.

During the final editing of the book manuscript I came across another article by Steven Lieberman. The headline was shocking, sad, but not surprising: "Rabbis who caused Evergreen Court fatal fire get plea with DA for no jail time."

As part of the deal, Nathaniel Sommer pleaded guilty to two counts of second-degree manslaughter, a felony, and is expected to be sentenced to five years' probation. His son, Aaron, pleaded guilty to one count of second-degree reckless endangerment, a misdemeanor, which carries a sentence of three years' probation. As part of the deal, Nathaniel Sommer pleaded guilty to two counts of second-degree manslaughter, a felony, and is expected to be sentenced to five years' probation. His son, Aaron, pleaded guilty to one count of second-degree reckless endangerment, a misdemeanor, which carries a sentence of three years' probation.

"He promised justice was going to be served," Davenport said of Walsh. "This deal is not justice."

Lloyd's mother, Sabrail Davenport, expressed her feelings about the plea in four words: "disappointment, disgusted, heartbroken, and betrayed."

She said Walsh told the family last week that this decision was in the best interest of the people.

"I asked him, 'What people? Not us,'" Davenport said, adding her son's life was lost for a probationary sentence and $600 in court fees.

After reading the article and adding portions to the manuscript, I felt the same as Sabrail Davenport did.[25]

---

25. lohud.com/story/news/local/rockland/spring-valley/
2023/06/20/evergreen-court-home-for-adults-fire-rabbiswho-
caused-fire-get-no-jail-in-plea-deal/70318690007/

BETSY'S CREATIVITY AND HOPE LETTERS

11

Overview

I never threw away most of the letters Betsy wrote to me. Each time I opened a letter or card, I rolled my eyes, took a deep breath, and sighed, because I never knew what to expect. After her death I was elated that some of her creative, sometimes happy, and thoughtful personality was saved.

A few more of Betsy's letters are included in this chapter, because they did not belong anywhere else in the book. Each one reflects the creativity and hope she had during the years of her illness. I do not know the month or year she wrote them, but I want her work to be read and remembered.

When She Wrote Her Letters

As noted previously, Betsy was often at her best when she was in the hospital, because she was working to get better and be discharged. During these times, she always wrote me a letter or two. She almost always went to the hospital when she was entering a severe manic state or when she needed to undergo tests. It is ironic that her last letter included her words of wisdom, which she was unable to follow. Although for years I tried to force normality where there wasn't normality, I always knew in my heart that she had to cope with living in a totally abnormal world. Her letters, written to me over the years, were blessings in disguise, because many of them are in this book.

The first letter is a summary of a book she had read; she wanted to share what she had learned with me. The second letter was written when she was in the Halifax Psychiatric Hospital in Daytona Beach, Florida. This letter was probably written to me in the early 1990s, because, based on my recollection, she lived in Daytona Beach during these years. My parents were living in Ormond Beach, which was about thirty minutes away.

God rest your dear soul, Betsy.

Dear Linsey + Frank,
   I read a book and outlined it. I'm
sending you a copy just to write and relax.

I)   Quotes

The first step toward success is identifying your own leadership
strengths. Teamwork ② Communication is built on trusting relationships ③ The first step toward success is identifying your own
leadership strengths ④ Motivation can never be forced. People have
to want to do a good job ⑤ There's nothing else more effective
and rewarding than showing a genuine interest in people ⑥ Step
outside yourself to discover what's imp't to someone else, ⑦ nothing
is more persuasive than a good listener. ⑧ Team players are
the leaders of tomorrow ⑨ Truly respecting others is the bedrock
of communication. ⑩ People work for money but go the extra mile
for recognition, praise and rewards ⑪ Set goals that are
clear, challenging and obtainable. ⑫ Be quick to admit mistakes and slow to criticize. Above all be constructive.
⑬ Consistently high performance comes from a balance between
work and leisure. Gain strength from the positive and don't be
sapped by the negative. ⑭ Tame your worries and energize
your life. ⑮ Never underestimate the power of enthusiasm

II) Discover how to:

① Identify your own leadership strengths ② build trusting relationships
③ Gain the respect you deserve ④ Eliminate the "us vs. them attitude
⑤ Achieve goals and increase self confidence ⑥ Become a flexible
risk taker ⑦ Solve problems more creatively ⑧ motivate yourself +
others ⑨ Listen more effectively to learn ⑩ Become a team
player and strengthen cooperation among associates ⑪ Improve
business and potential relationships ⑪ Think and communicate
more clearly ⑫ Change your attitude toward mistakes ⑬ Balance

The Human Relations Revolution
   ① Finding the Leader in You ② Starting to communicate
③ Motivating People ④ Expressing genuine Interest in people
④ Seeing things from the other's point of view ⑤ Motivating peo
⑥ Listening to learn ⑦ Teaming up for tomorrow ⑧ Respecting the
dignity of others ⑨ Recognition, praise and rewards ⑩ Heading
mistakes, complaints and criticisms ⑪ Setting goals ⑫ Focus on
principles ⑬ Achieving balance ⑭ Creating a positive mental attitude
⑮ Learning not to worry

Conclusion : making it happen.

- be here now, in this moment
respect your unique self
attend to joy
use self discipline as a road
to wisdom
incorporate balance and rhythm
in living
live simply and freely
be involved in self-creation

I'm writing these self-help
ideas because I know

_____

Again —

Happy Anniversary

♡

I need your advice
on my love life.

Love,
Me

Dear Linsey,
when you don't feel
well reward yourself. Take
long, hot, scented bath. Read
novel, go to a movie with
someone special, listen to
music. Read poetry, shop,
out w/ friends, nature, a
marriage, a museum, a
cail. Browse in a bookstore
antique shop, pet shop, boo
Stress: don't overdo it. understa
you aren't running because yo
in a hurry to get somewhere

Anyway, you can help
me w/ a call these
next few weeks. I kno
I ask alot but I
really would like
flowers — everybody el
gets them. My address

Betsy ....
Halifax Psychiatric Cente

BIBLIOGRAPHY

Alderman, Time, "The Forgotten Story of Rosemary Kennedy, Who Was Lobotomized So That JFK Could Succeed." All That's Interesting, last updated May 2, 2022. https://allthatsinteresting.com/rosemary-kennedy.

American Psychiatric Association. "Frequently Asked Questions." American Psychiatric Association (website), accessed date of access. https://www.psychiatry.org/psychiatrists/practice/dsm/frequently-asked-questions.

Castelluccio, M. "'You Want to See Him Again': 1 Year after Evergreen Court Fire, Lloyd's Loss, Questions Linger." Preserve Ramapo, March 23, 2022. https://preserve-ramapo.com/you-want-to-see-him-again-1-year-after-evergreen-court-fire-lloyds-loss-questions-linger/.

Dembosky, April, Amelia Templeton, and Carrie Feibel. "When Homelessness and Mental Illness Overlap, Is Forced Treatment Compassionate?" NPR, March 31, 2023. https://www.npr.org/sections/health-shots/2023/03/31/1164281917/when-homelessness-and-mental-illness-overlap-is-compulsory-treatment-compassiona.

Larson, Zeb. "Don't Bring Back Mental Asylums. Instead, Build the Welfare State." Jacobin, March 8, 2023. https://jacobin.com/2023/03/mental-asylums-welfare-state-involuntary-incarceration-hospitalization.

Lieberman, Steve. (June 20, 2023). "Rabbis who Caused Evergreen Court Fatal Fire Get Plea With DA for No Jail Time." *Rockland/Westchester Journal News*, June 20, 2023.

Lieberman, Steve. (February 2, 2023). "Evergreen Court Fire: Charges against Former Spring Valley Building Inspector Dismissed." *Rockland Westchester Journal News,* February 2, 2023.

Lieberman, Steve. "Evergreen Court Fire Victim's Sons Sue Facility, Others over His Death: What to Know." *Rockland/Westchester Journal News*, November 23, 2022.

Lieberman, Steve. "Evergreen Court Rabbis Ask Judge to Dismiss Indictment," *Rockland/Westchester Journal News*, June 27, 2022.

Lieberman, Steve. "Evergreen Fire: Felony Counts Against Rabbis in Fatal Adult Home Inferno Upheld." *Rockland/Westchester Journal News*, September 14, 2022.

Lieberman, Steve. "Evergreen Fire: Will Rabbis' Indictment Stand? Here's What Judge Is Deciding." *Rockland/Westchester Journal News*, September 6, 2022.

Lieberman, Steve. (September 7, 2022). "Jared Lloyd's Mom Files Wrongful Death Lawsuit against Spring Valley Rabbis and Others." *Rockland/Westchester Journal News*, September 7, 2022.

Mental Health America. "The State of Mental Health in America." Mental Health America (website), 2023. https://mhanational.org/issues/state-mental-health-america.

National Alliance for the Mentally Ill. Brochure. 1993.

National Institute of Mental Health. "Mental Illness," National Institute of Mental Health (website), last updated March 2023. https://www.nimh.nih.gov/health/statistics/mental-illness.

The New York Times Editorial Board. "The Solution to America's Mental Health Crisis Already Exists," *The New York Times*, October 4, 2022, https://www.nytimes.com/2022/10/04/opinion/us-mental-health-community-centers.html.

Nirmita Panchal, Heather Saunders, Robin Rudowitz, and Cynthia Cox, "The Implications of COVID-19 for Mental Health and Substance Use," KFF, March 20, 2023, https://www.kff.org/coronavirus-covid-19/issue-brief/the-implications-of-covid-19-for-mental-health-and-substance-use/.

"Rosemary Kennedy." Wikipedia, last updated May 6, 2023. https://en.wikipedia.org/wiki/Rosemary_Kennedy.

Simpson, Mona. "America Has No Way to Take Care of Mentally Ill People." *Time,* March 23, 2023. https://time.com/6265241/america-care-of-mentally-ill-people/.

"The Solution to America's Mental Health Crisis Already Exists," Editorial. *New York Times,* October 2, 2022.

Truschel, Jessica. "Bipolar Definition and DSM-5 Diagnostic Criteria." Remedy Health Media, LLC. September 29, 2020, https://www.psycom.net/bipolar-definition-dsm-5.

Welber, Bobby. "Massive Fire at Mid-Hudson Region Nursing Home Kills at Least 1." *Hudson Valley Post, March 23, 2021.*

World Health Organization. "COVID-19 Pandemic Triggers 25% Increase in Prevalence of Anxiety and Depression Worldwide." World Health Organization (website), March 2, 2022. https://www.who.int/news/item/02-03-2022-covid-19-pandemic-triggers-25-increase-in-prevalence-of-anxiety-and-depression-worldwide.

SUGGESTED READING

Adam, David. *The Man Who Couldn't Stop: OCD and the True Story of a Life Lost in Thought.* New York: Picador, 2016.

Allen, Sandy. *A Kind of Miraculous Paradise: A True Story about Schizophrenia.* New York: Scribner, 2018.

Benincasa, Sara. *Dispatches from My Bedroom with Agorafabulous.* New York: William Morrow & Company, 2013.

Burroughs, Augusten. *Running with Scissors: A Memoir.* New York: Picador, 2002.

Cahalan, Susannah. *Brain on Fire: My Month of Madness.* New York: Simon and Schuster, 2013.

Casey, Neil, ed. *Unholy Ghost: Writers on Depression.* New York: Morrow, 2001.

Charlamagne tha God. *Shook One: Anxiety Playing Tricks on Me.* New York: Atria Books, 2019.

Cheney, Terri. *Manic: A Memoir.* New York: William Morrow, 2008.

Colas, Emily. *Just Checking: Scenes from the Life of an Obsessive Compulsive.* New York: Washington Square Press, 1998.

Danquah, Meri Nana-Ama. *Willow Weep for Me: A Black Woman's Journey through Depression.* New York: W.W. Norton & Company, 1998.

Forney, Ellen. *Marbles: Mania, Depression, Michelangelo, and Me; A Graphic Memoir.* New York: Gotham Books, 2012.

Hamilton, Suzy Favor. *Fast Girl: A Life Spent Running from Madness.* New York: Dey Street Books, 2015.

Hazzard, Vanessa, Iresha Picot, and Rasheedah Phillips, eds. *The Color of Hope: People of Color Mental Health Narratives.* North Charleston, SC: CreateSpace Independent Publishing Platform, 2015.

Jamison, Kay R. *An Unquiet Mind: A Memoir of Moods and Madness.* New York: Vintage Books/Random House, 1995.

Jensen, Kelly, ed. *(Don't) Call Me Crazy: 33 Voices Start the Conversation about Mental Health.* Chapel Hill, NC: Algonquin Young Readers/Algonquin Books, 2018.

Karr, Mary. *Lit: A Memoir.* New York: Harper, 2009.

Khakpour, Porochista. *Sick: A Memoir.* New York: Harper Perennial, 2018.

LaPera, Amanda. *Losing Dad: Paranoid Schizophrenia; A Family's Search for Hope.* Aliso Viejo, CA: Adamo Press, 2013.

LeFavour, Cree. *Lights On, Rats Out: A Memoir.* New York: Grove Press, 2017.

Lowe, Jaime. *Mental: Lithium, Love, and Losing My Mind.* New York: Blue Rider Press/Penguin Random House, 2017.

Mailhot, Terese Marie. *Heart Berries: A Memoir.* Berkeley, CA: Counterpoint, 2018.

McClelland, Mac. *Irritable Hearts: A PTSD Love Story.* New York: Flatiron Books, 2015.

McDaniels, Darryl. *Ten Ways Not to Commit Suicide.* New York: Amistad, 2016.

Merkin, Daphne. *This Close to Happy: A Reckoning with Depression.* New York: Farrar, Straus, and Giroux, 2017.

Moezzi, Melody. *Haldol and Hyacinths: A Bipolar Life.* New York: Avery, 2014.

Pershall, Stacy. *Loud in the House of Myself: Memoir of a Strange Girl.* New York: W.W. Norton & Company, 2011.

Pierce-Baker, Charlotte. *This Fragile Life: A Mother's Story of a Bipolar Son.* Chicago: Lawrence Hill Books, 2012.

Ramprasad, Gayathri. *Shadows in the Sun: Healing from Depression and Finding the Light Within.* Center City, MN: Hazelden Publishing, 2014.

Saks, Elyn R. *The Center Cannot Hold: My Journey through Madness.* New York: Hyperion, 2007.

Schiller, Lori, and Amanda Bennett. *The Quiet Room: A Journey out of the Torment of Madness.* New York: Grand Central Publishing, 1994.

Shields, Brooke. *Down Came the Rain: My Journey through Postpartum Depression.* New York: Hyperion, 2005.

Solomon, Andrew. *The Noonday Demon: An Atlas of Depression.* New York: Scribner, 2001.

Stossel, Scott. *My Age of Anxiety: Fear, Hope, Dread, and the Search for Peace of Mind.* New York: Vintage Books, 2015.

Styron, William. *Darkness Visible: A Memoir of Madness.* New York: Random House, 1990.

Talusan, Grace. *The Body Papers: A Memoir.* New York: Restless Books, 2019.

Van Gelder, Kiera. *The Buddha & the Borderline: My Recovery from Borderline Personality Disorder through Dialectical*

Behavior Therapy, Buddhism, & Online Dating. Oakland, CA: New Harbinger Publications, 2010.

Vonnegut, Mark, MD. *Just Like Someone without Mental Illness Only More So: A Memoir.* New York: Delacorte Press, 2010.

Wang, Esmé Weijun. *The Collected Schizophrenias.* Minneapolis, MN: Graywolf Press, 2019.

Washuta, Elissa. *My Body is a Book of Rules.* Pasadena, CA: Red Hen Press, 2014.

Wurtzel, Elizabeth. *Prozac Nation: Young and Depressed in Americs: A Memoir.* New York: Riverhead Books, 1994.

ABOUT THE AUTHOR

Linsey Willis, D.P.A., SPHR, is an author with forty-four years of Human Resources experience as a management and organizational consultant, expert witness, coach, and educator. Dr. Willis' multi-faceted experience includes service to clients in private sector, city, county, state, and federal government agencies and companies in the US and internationally. Her previous publications include *Mastering the Assessment Center Process*, published in 2017. *Developing Your Innate Abilities* was written to help college students and those seeking promotions develop their soft skills.

Her passion for excellence and dedication to developing leadership qualities in others have served people in many ways, including: police personnel who have been promoted to management ranks throughout the US; college students who have received stipends from her book royalty fund (established at Florida Atlantic University's College of Business); and court cases where she was an expert witness have been settled.

ACKNOWLEDGMENTS

I started writing this book in or around 1990, well over 30 years ago. The first draft was a labor of love, pain and a process of catharsis. From the beginning, I have had the full support of our parents. After reading the first draft my mother commented that I was a bit critical of my father. However, after having perused the draft he never appeared upset or stated his disagreement. He also believed it would be worthy of publication after completion and editing. From my dear husband, Frank, I had learned to always retain my files. Saving the early versions was one of the best decisions I could have made because building on them, I was able to complete the book and take it to publication. Needless to say, I never expected that Betsy's life would end the way it did.

Primarily, I thank my wonderful parents Joan and Bob Craig (both deceased) for supporting and encouraging me when I completed the first very rough draft. They said that if I ever finished the book they believed it would be published. I believe they would have been pleased and proud of the publication of our family's story. My husband, Frank, also deserves many heartfelt thanks because through the good and bad times, he has always been present for me. He witnessed and experienced many horrible and very sad situations with Betsy but was always calm, positive and attentive. He has always been a great listener and is my "Rock of Gibraltar."

Drs. Robert S. Sloat and Erica Goodstone, two long term and dear friends, played instrumental roles in the process of editing my book before I submitted it to many book publishers. Bob has been a long term associate for my consulting business and is a very good editor and confidant. His experience writing many published journal articles when he was a university professor at several universities and colleges was very beneficial. Erica's contributions were also very significant as well as interesting. She too has published many articles, and books. Overall, their comments and suggestions resulted in an improved reading experience. I was so touched when Bob told me that while he was reading the book he cried. His wife Beth, a fine artist, medical graphic artist and teacher, with a BA in English, made some valuable comments and edits to the first few chapters.

Dr. Christopher Fichera has been my therapist for more than 20 years and has always listened attentively when I share stories about my life and Betsy's life. He has helped me build my self-esteem. Dr. Fichera was extremely encouraging and supportive during the several months after Betsy's death when I was finishing this book. His support facilitated the momentum I needed to keep going particularly because he felt strongly that the book would be published and purchased. Thank you so much Dr. Fichera.

Brenda and Alan Zuniss, two long-term and dear friends, had met Betsy on a few occasions and were understanding, empathetic and non-judgmental about her condition. You read about them in the book and they were with me during my last social visit with Betsy. They wanted to ensure that we all had a pleasant and successful visit. For example, they wanted to make sure that we found a hair salon in Haverstraw, NY where she could have a haircut before we took her to lunch. Diane Stevens, a dear friend whom I met at Rotary club in downtown Boca Raton, Florida, has also been very supportive and understanding about my sister's plight and how I was handling it. You read about what she and her husband Bill contributed to Betsy and the other victims of the fire in Spring Valley, NY.

I decided to design the draft cover for the book and then submit it to Amplify Publishing. After the staff at Amplify sent me their versions, I decided that I was not happy with any of mine or theirs. Simultaneously, I called my high school friend Patty Sanders, who I have stayed in touch with over the years and asked for her opinion. The only image she thought was just okay was a black and white drawing of the face of a person with bipolar illness. Then I had an "AHA" moment and asked if her sister Sue Miller was still doing artwork. I remembered that one subject of her art was paintings of family members. Patty said "yes" and told me to share my ideas with Susie, asking if she could paint a picture of a face depicting the depressed and manic phases. We scheduled a phone call where the three of us discussed all of the cover versions. She asked me if I could send a very old color picture of Betsy to her with which she could work. The picture was of Betsy in her late teens or early twenties when she was beautiful and vibrant. Sue used it for the painting which cannot be described by just one word. My own reactions and those of a few other friends included: "formidable, impressive, outstanding, gorgeous, wow, amazing, and that the picture talks to you". Thank you so much Sue for your wonderful work. I loved collaborating with you and seeing the painting develop from beginning to end. I believe that the cover will help sell the book. Thank you too, Patty, for taking a few hours of your time to collaborate with us.

Even before the publication of this book, I had many visions of seeing the book on the shelves in the airport shops nestled in between other new releases or bestsellers. After the cover was completed, when I was traveling the fall of 2023, I visited some airport shops and seeing the new releases and bestseller signs, I envisioned passersby first noticing a vibrant, startling and beautiful book cover, then stopping to read the title, opening the book to the table of contents, flipping through a few pages and then walking to the register and purchasing it. Thank you again, Sue.

I also acknowledge several other friends who were very supportive and interested when I told them about the book and when I completed it. I use only their first names to protect their privacy: Paul, Chris, Alan, Brigette, two Dianes, and Karina.

Finally, the publication of this book would not have been possible had Lauren Magnussen, Director of Production, not selected it from the hundreds of submissions Amplify receives each year. She was very supportive, encouraging, enthusiastic, and totally engaged in the process. She told me that the book was timely and that many people would benefit from reading it.